HIV/AIDS Primary Care Handbook

HIV/AIDS Primary Care Handbook

Cynthia G. Carmichael, MD
Assistant Clinical Professor
Department of Family Medicine & Community Health
University of Miami School of Medicine
Miami, Florida

J. Kevin Carmichael, MD
Assistant Clinical Professor
Department of Family & Community Medicine
University of Arizona College of Medicine

Unit Chief, El Rio Special Immunology Associates
El Rio Community Health Center
Tucson, Arizona

Margaret A. Fischl, MD
Professor, Department of Medicine
Director, Comprehensive AIDS Program
University of Miami School of Medicine
Miami, Florida

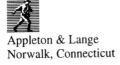

Appleton & Lange
Norwalk, Connecticut

ISBN: 0-8385-3557-7

Notice: The authors and the publisher of this volume have taken care to make certain that the doses of drugs and schedules of treatment are correct and compatible with the standards generally accepted at the time of publication. Nevertheless, as new information becomes available, changes in treatment and in the use of drugs become necessary. The reader is advised to carefully consult the instruction and information material included in the package insert of each drug or therapeutic agent before administration. This advice is especially important when using new and infrequently used drugs. The publisher disclaims any liability, loss, injury, or damage incurred as a consequence, directly or indirectly, of the use and application of any of the contents of this volume.

Copyright © 1995 by Appleton & Lange
A Simon & Schuster Company

All rights reserved. This book, or any parts thereof, may not be used or reproduced in any manner without written permission. For information, address Appleton & Lange, 25 Van Zant Street, East Norwalk, Connecticut 06855.

95 96 97 98 99 / 10 9 8 7 6 5 4 3 2 1

Prentice Hall International (UK) Limited, *London*
Prentice Hall of Australia Pty. Limited, *Sydney*
Prentice Hall Canada, Inc., *Toronto*
Prentice Hall Hispanoamericana, S.A., *Mexico*
Prentice Hall of India Private Limited, *New Delhi*
Prentice Hall of Japan, Inc., *Tokyo*
Simon and Schuster Asia Pte. Ltd., *Singapore*
Editora Prentice Hall do Brasil Ltda., *Rio de Janeiro*
Prentice Hall, *Englewood Cliffs, New Jersey*

ISSN: 1077-3517

Cover illustration: Electronic micrograph of HIV-infected lymphocytes. Reproduced with permission from Brooks GF, Butel JS, & Ornston LN: *Jawetz, Melnick & Adelberg's Medical Microbiology*, 19th ed., Appleton & Lange, 1991

Acquisitions Editor: Shelley Reinhardt
Production Editor: Elizabeth C. Ryan
Designer: Michael J. Kelly

PRINTED IN THE UNITED STATES OF AMERICA

Contents

Contributors..vii
Preface ix

1. The State of the Epidemic 1
2. HIV Testing 5
3. An Overview of HIV Care 11
4. Initial Patient Visit...13
5. Follow-up Examination 19
6. Prophylaxis Against Opportunistic Infections....................23
7. Antiretroviral Therapy & Strategy 33
8. Common HIV-Associated Infections & Conditions..........45
9. Differential Diagnosis of Common Complaints
   in HIV-Infected Individuals...93

10. HIV Infection in Women 107

11. HIV Infection in Children 119

12. HIV & Nutrition 133
*Richard S. Beach, MD, PhD, &
Cynthia A. Thomson, MS, RD, CNSD*

13. Experimental & Nontraditional Treatments for AIDS 147

14. Health Care Workers & HIV 151

15. Medications Commonly Used in
HIV-Infected Individuals 157
*Cindy M. Maggio, PharmD,
Kimberley J. Campbell, PharmD, RPh,
Mary Greene Manning, PharmD,
Michael D. Katz, PharmD,
Teresa C. Nord, PharmD, & Kari A. Wieland, PharmD*

Appendix

- 1993 Revised Classification for HIV Infection &
  Expanded Surveillance Case Definition for AIDS
  Among Adolescents & Adults 202
- Classification of HIV Infection in Children
  Under 13 Years of Age 204
- Adult HIV/AIDS Confidential Case Report Form 207
- TMP/SMX Desensitization Protocol 209
- Patient Instructions for TMP/SMX
  Desensitization 211
- Mental Status Examination 212
- Florida Living Will & Authorization 214
- Resources for Practitioners & Patients 216

Index 219

Detachable Pocket Medication Card

Contributors

Richard S. Beach, MD, PhD
Medical Director, Comprehensive Pediatrics AIDS Program, Fort Lauderdale; Physician in private practice, Comprehensive Immune Care, Miami Beach, Florida.

Kimberley J. Campbell, PharmD, RPh
Research Specialist, University of Arizona Cancer Center, Tucson, Arizona.

Cynthia G. Carmichael, MD
Assistant Clinical Professor, Department of Family Medicine & Community Health, University of Miami School of Medicine, Miami, Florida.

J. Kevin Carmichael, MD
Assistant Clinical Professor, Department of Family & Community Medicine, University of Arizona College of Medicine; Unit Chief, El Rio Special Immunology Associates, El Rio Community Health Center, Tucson, Arizona.

Margaret A. Fischl, MD
Professor, Department of Medicine; Director, Comprehensive AIDS Program, University of Miami School of Medicine, Miami, Florida.

Michael D. Katz, PharmD
Associate Professor, Department of Pharmacy Practice, University of Arizona College of Pharmacy, Tucson, Arizona.

Cindy M. Maggio, PharmD
Clinical Pharmacist—Special Immunology, Department of Pharmacy, Department of Veterans Affairs, Miami, Florida.

Mary Greene Manning, PharmD
Clinical Pharmacist, Scottsdale Memorial Hospital-North; Adjunct Faculty, University of Arizona College of Pharmacy, Scottsdale, Arizona.

Teresa C. Nord, PharmD
Associate in Pharmacy Practice, Tucson Medical Center, Tucson, Arizona.

Cynthia A. Thomson, MS, RD, CNSD
Clinical Nutrition Research Specialist, Department of Family & Community Medicine, University of Arizona College of Medicine, Tucson, Arizona.

Kari A. Wieland, PharmD
Clinical Ambulatory Care Specialist, Veterans Affairs Medical Center, Reno; Clinical Assistant Professor, University of Nevada School of Medicine, Reno; Adjunct Clinical Professor, Idaho State University School of Pharmacy, Reno, Nevada.

Preface

This book began as an effort to provide guidelines regarding HIV/AIDS care for physicians practicing in community health centers in South Florida. Annual revisions over the last five years (with the support of the Dade County Area Health Education Center and the Florida AIDS Education and Training Center) have resulted in the text presented here.

Caring for people with HIV infection challenges health care providers and society at many levels. The amount of new information and rapid change in clinical practice often results in a lack of consensus in the literature and among experts. Our goal in this text is to interpret the current data and make suggestions that are as clinically relevant and concise as possible. We will continue to update this text annually and welcome your comments.

Despite the tragedies of this epidemic, we have been fortunate to witness the heroism of our patients and their friends and families, as well as the compassion of our co-workers. Furthermore, we are grateful for the loving support of our families in our work.

We dedicate this book to hope.

Cynthia G. Carmichael, MD
J. Kevin Carmichael, MD
Margaret A. Fischl, MD

ACKNOWLEDGMENTS

We gratefully acknowledge the following individuals for their thoughtful review of various sections of the manuscript:

Neil Ampel, MD
Associate Professor of Medicine
University of Arizona Health Sciences Center
Tucson Veterans Affairs Medical Center

Joseph Berger, MD
Professor
Department of Neurology
University of Miami School of Medicine

David Fink, MD
Community Physician
Miami Beach

Andrew Helfgott, MD
Assistant Professor
Division of Maternal-Fetal Medicine
Department of Obstetrics & Gynecology
University of Miami School of Medicine

Mary Jo O'Sullivan, MD
Professor & Chief
Division of Maternal-Fetal Medicine
Department of Obstetrics & Gynecology
University of Miami School of Medicine

Arthur Pitchenik, MD
Professor
Pulmonary Division
Department of Medicine
University of Miami School of Medicine
Veterans Affairs Medical Center, Miami

Gwendolyn Scott, MD
Professor & Director
Division of Pediatric Infectious Diseases & Immunology
Department of Pediatrics
University of Miami School of Medicine

Paula Sparti, MD
Community Physician
Miami

Raj Uttamchandani, MD
Community Physician
Miami

1
The State of the Epidemic

Acquired immunodeficiency syndrome (AIDS) cases in the world number more than 2,600,000. There are an estimated 12.9 million HIV-infected people (8 million in Africa).

AIDS cases in the United States number 339,250 (57% deceased). An estimated 1 million people are HIV-infected (1 in every 250 adults).

CURRENT TRENDS IN THE UNITED STATES

Mode of Infection: In 1992, a little over one-half of the reported AIDS cases were among men with homosexual/bisexual contacts. However, the number of cases reported from this group has decreased during the past 2 years.

Cases associated with injecting-drug use (IDU) increased slightly in 1992.

Cases attributed to heterosexual contact jumped 17.1% from 1991 with 59.4% of those being women. As would follow, cases resulting from perinatal transmission also increased during 1992.

Gender: In 1992, women comprised 14.1% of reported AIDS cases. Over 50% of these women came from 10 metropolitan areas. The modes of infection for these women varied by geographic region with IDU predominating in the northeast and heterosexual transmission equaling or surpassing IDU elsewhere.

Age: The reported number of AIDS cases in the age range of 20–29 years has increased 15.5% since 1988. This primarily reflects individuals infected as adolescents. In the past two years, the number of 13- to 21-year-olds who have become HIV-infected in the USA has increased by 77%.

From 1988 to 1992, a national seroprevalence survey of Job Corps students (ages 16–21) found that 1 in every 278 students is HIV-infected; young women have a higher prevalence than young men.

In 1992, HIV became the leading cause of death for men between the ages of 25 and 44 in the USA; for women ages 25–44, HIV was the fourth leading cause of death. It has been estimated that by the year 1995 there will be 45,600 children and adolescents orphaned by maternal deaths caused by HIV/AIDS.

Race/Ethnicity: In 1992, the majority (47.4%) of reported AIDS cases were among white, non-Hispanic individuals. Among women, however, rates were higher for non-Hispanic blacks and Hispanics than for non-Hispanic whites.

Socioeconomic status among other factors, no doubt, figure into the overall incidence of AIDS being higher in the non-Hispanic black and Hispanic populations than in the white, non-Hispanic population.

Note: AIDS cases are reported to the Centers for Disease Control and Prevention (CDC) via local health departments. See the Appendix for the 1993 Revised Classification for HIV Infection and Expanded Surveillance Case Definition for AIDS Among Adolescents and Adults and for the CDC confidential case report form. At this time, the federal government requests voluntary physician cooperation in AIDS case reporting. However, many state and local authorities not only mandate AIDS reporting, but also positive HIV test results (Table 1–1). Failure to report these results may result in penalties or loss of medical license.

TABLE 1–1. HUMAN IMMUNODEFICIENCY VIRUS INFECTION—REPORTING REQUIREMENTS

By Name	Anonymous	Not Required
Alabama	Georgia	Alaska
Arizona	Iowa	California
Arkansas	Kansas	Connecticut
Colorado	Kentucky	Delaware
Idaho	Maine	Florida
Illinois	Montana	Hawaii
Indiana	New Hampshire	Louisiana
Michigan	Oregon	Maryland*
Minnesota	Rhode Island	Massachusetts
Mississippi	Texas	Nebraska
Missouri		New Mexico
Nevada		New York
New Jersey		Pensylvania
North Carolina		Vermont
North Dakota		Washington*
Ohio		District of Colombia
Oklahoma		
South Carolina		
South Dakota		
Tennessee		
Utah		
Virginia		
West Virginia		
Wisconsin		
Wyoming		

*Symptomatic HIV infection must be reported by name
From: Centers for Disease Control. Public health user of HIV-infection reports—South Carolina, 1986–1991. MMWR 1992;41:245.

REFERENCES

Centers for Disease Control and Prevention. HIV/AIDS Surveillance Report, 1993;5 (no.3) Data through September 1993.

Conway G, Epstein MR, Hayman CR et al: Trends in HIV prevalence among disadvantaged youth: Survey results from a national job training program, 1988–1992. *JAMA* 1993;**269:**2887.

Goldsmith MF: "Invisible" epidemic now becoming visible as HIV/AIDS pandemic reaches adolescents. *JAMA* 1993;**270:**16.

Karon JM, Doncero TJ, Curran JW: The projected incidence of AIDS and estimated prevalence of HIV infection in the United States. *J Acquir Immune Defic Syndr* 1988;**1:**542.

Mann JM, Tarantola DJM, Netter T (editors): *AIDS in the World.* Harvard Univ Press, 1992.

Michaels D, Levine C: Estimates of the number of motherless youth orphaned by AIDS in the United States. *JAMA* 1992;**268:**3456.

Centers for Disease Control and Prevention. Update: Acquired Immunodeficiency Syndrome—United States, 1992. *MMWR* 1993;**42:**547.

Centers for Disease Control and Prevention. Update: Mortality Attributable to HIV infection among persons aged 25–44 years—United States, 1991 and 1992. *MMWR* 1993;**42:**869.

2
HIV Testing

HIV infection is now the leading cause of death for young men and among the leading causes of death for young women in the USA. Yet, studies reveal that HIV seropositive individuals often learn of their infection only *after* they develop an opportunistic infection or other serious HIV-related condition. Furthermore, in one anonymous screening study in an urban emergency department, 65% of the identified seropositive individuals had unrecognized infection. The National AIDS Behavioral Surveys (NABS) found that over 60% of those individuals at highest risk for HIV infection had never had an HIV test.

HIV RISK ASSESSMENT

Primary care practitioners are in an excellent position to educate, assess risk, and encourage HIV testing for their patients. A recent report noted, however, that while 94% of physicians surveyed routinely asked their patients about cigarette smoking, only 22–49% of those physicians inquired about specific sexual behaviors and practices. A substantial number of physicians are missing opportunities to educate their patients about HIV and test patients for infection.

A brief discussion of HIV and its transmission is recommended with all patients. Certain behaviors place some individuals at higher risk of exposure to HIV than others; however, given the changing epidemiology of this disease, screening of all patients and offering the HIV test is the responsibility of the attentive primary care physician.

Following are five questions for HIV risk assessment:

1. Did you receive a transfusion of blood products between 1978 and 1985?
2. Have you ever, even once, used any recreational drugs (includes injected drugs and crack cocaine)?
3. Have you had any form of sex in the past 5 years?
4. Have you ever had a sexually transmitted disease?
5. Have you ever had tuberculosis?

These questions serve to introduce a more detailed discussion of HIV. In addition, they may stimulate patients to carefully consider past and present circumstances and behaviors.

There are many benefits of learning one's HIV status. For infected individuals, it presents the opportunities for antiretroviral therapy, opportunistic infection prophylaxis, prevention of HIV transmission to others, tuberculosis screening and chemoprophylaxis (if indicated). Preventive immunizations and medical monitoring may delay onset of AIDS and prolong life.

PRETEST COUNSELING

Prior to HIV testing, the CDC recommends—and many states mandate—pretest counseling. Counseling should be "client-centered" and sensitive to the cultural values and sexual identity of the individual. In addition, counseling should be developmentally appropriate for the individual's age and learning skills and consistent with the individual's language, dialect, terminology, and style of communication.

Counseling and testing of adolescents requires understanding age-specific development and behavior patterns, such as emerging sexuality, feelings of invulnerability, and experimentation with risk-taking behaviors. Assessing the individual's ability to cope, to comprehend, and to give informed consent for the test is essential. Visual demonstrations, repetition, and explicit language help reinforce provided information. Young women in particular may need to learn, discuss, and practice negotiating latex condom use with their sexual partners.

Pretest counseling should include:

1. Providing detailed information on HIV, AIDS, and transmission of HIV.
2. Describing behaviors that put a patient at risk for HIV exposure.
3. Discussing methods to reduce risk of exposure, including use of latex condoms. Be aware that for certain highly vulnerable women, their suggesting condom use has been linked to an increased risk of violence.
4. Discussing possible obstacles to adopting risk-reduction practices.
5. Clarifying the meaning of a negative HIV test result (patient is not immune from HIV and must protect him or herself).
6. Clarifying the meaning of a positive HIV test result (patient may transmit HIV infection to others).
7. Clarifying the meaning of false positive, and indeterminate results.
8. Discussing the availability of anonymous testing, confidentiality of test results, and state reporting laws.
9. Inquiring how the patient will cope in the event of a positive test. The potential impact on employment, housing, health insurance, and possible ramifications concerning these issues should also be discussed.
10. Asking the patient to identify someone with whom test results may be discussed. This is particularly important for adolescents.
11. Obtaining consent (be informed of local statutes regarding testing of minors).
12. Making arrangements for a return appointment to receive test results.

HIV TESTS

A diagnosis of HIV infection is based on the presence of antibodies to HIV-1 in the blood. In most individuals, antibody develops within 6–12 weeks after infection. During the initial 6–12 weeks after infection—the window period—the enzyme-linked immunosorbent assay (ELISA) HIV antibody test will be negative. An individual is considered HIV positive only after a blood sample tests positive by ELISA, and is confirmed by either a positive Western blot or indirect immunofluorescent assay (IFA).

Although the ELISA is a sensitive screening test, some false-positive results do occur. Reactive ELISA tests require confirmation with a Western blot or equivalent test, such as the IFA.

The Western blot involves separation of individual viral proteins into defined bands. The presence of any two of the p-24, gp41, or gp 120/160 bands, designate a positive Western blot. An "indeterminate" result means the blood does not meet the two-band requirement, but does show some of the bands characteristic of HIV-1.

Indeterminate test results may occur in individuals with early HIV-1 infection, HIV-2 (a related retrovirus infection found in some individuals from West Africa or the Caribbean), or in healthy uninfected individuals (true false-positives). Indeterminate test results should be repeated in 3–6 months or followed with an HIV-2 antibody test if clinically indicated.

Antigen testing for the p-24 antigen may be useful in detecting early infection in the "window period," although this antigen may not always be present. Polymerase chain reaction [PCR] and viral culture are discussed in Chapter 11, "HIV in Children."

Office-based HIV testing is available, however, the use of a qualified laboratory with the capacity for confirmatory testing is recommended. Saliva HIV tests are being evaluated.

POSTTEST COUNSELING

Posttest counseling is imperative, regardless of the test result. It provides an opportunity to discuss risk-reducing behaviors with both seropositive and seronegative patients.

Practitioners must be aware of state laws on HIV and AIDS reporting and issues of confidentiality.

Posttest counseling should include:

1. Giving test results and explaining that a negative result does not imply immunity to infection, and explaining that a positive result means that the individual is infected and infectious.
2. Reviewing routes of transmission and risk-reduction strategies.
3. Assessing the patient's understanding of the test result and their psychological state. Involve the support person (see No. 10 under "Pretest Counseling," above) as necessary.
4. Providing psychologic support and referring to social service support organizations.
5. Providing information on national and local HIV/AIDS resources if indicated.
6. Providing referrals for medical follow-up and beginning to develop an individual medical care plan for the patient.
7. Discussing the importance of notifying needle-sharing or sexual partners, and the option of contact-tracing (as per local health department). Be sensitive to the risk of violence to women that may result from partner notification.

PREVENTION

The purpose of HIV testing is two-fold:

- To identify infected individuals so they can receive appropriate medical and preventive intervention
- To educate both HIV seropositive and seronegative individuals about prevention of further transmission of the virus

A full discussion of HIV screening and prevention in the USA and elsewhere is beyond the scope of this book. Proposals for screening have included a recommendation that routine voluntary testing of all inpatients between 15–54 years of age be offered at hospitals with an AIDS-diagnosis rate of 1 or more per 1,000 discharges per year. This cost-effective strategy would identify 68% of all HIV-infected patients admitted with conditions other than AIDS.

Increased HIV screening must be linked to enhanced and expanded medical and preventive services in order to care for newly identified patients.

REFERENCES

American Medical Association: HIV blood test counseling: AMA physician guidelines. 1988. American Medical Association.

Berrios D et al: HIV antibody testing among those at risk for infection: The national AIDS behavioral surveys. *JAMA* 1993;**270:**1576.

Bresolin L, Rinaldi R: Human immunodeficiency virus blood test counseling for adolescents. *Arch Fam Med* 1993;**2:**673.

Center for Disease Control and Prevention. HIV prevention practices of primary-care physicians—United States, 1992. *MMWR* 1994;**42:**988.

Center for Disease Control. Public Health Service guidelines for counseling and antibody testing to prevent HIV infection and AIDS. *MMWR* 1987;**36:**509.

Francis D: Toward a comprehensive HIV prevention program for the CDC and the nation. *JAMA* 1992;**268:**1444.

Goldschmidt RH: Laboratory testing for the presence of HIV infection and the progression of HIV disease. *JABFP* 1990;**3:**60.

Janssen R et al: HIV infection among patients in US acute care hospitals: Strategies for the counseling and testing of hospital patients. *N Engl J Med* 1992;**327:**447.

Kelen GD et al: Human immunodeficiency virus infection in emergency department patients: epidemiology, clinical presentations, and risk to health care workers: The Johns Hopkins experience. *JAMA* 1989;**262:**516.

North R, Rothenberg K: Partner notification and the threat of domestic violence against women with HIV infection. *N Engl J Med* 1993;**329:**1194.

Quinn TC: Screening for HIV infection—benefits and costs. *N Engl J Med* 1992;**327:**486.

Sloand E et al: HIV testing: State of the art. *JAMA* 1991;**266:**2861.

3
An Overview of HIV Care

Five key components of HIV care include:

1. Prevention of transmission
   Attention to risk factor assessment and active counseling toward risk reduction is essential.
2. Preservation of immune function
   Preservation of immune function is primarily a function of antiretroviral therapy. Increasing evidence suggests, however, that a "healthy lifestyle" and attention to adequate nutrition may also preserve immune function.
3. Prophylaxis against opportunistic infection
   Prophylaxis against *Pneumocystis carinii* pneumonia (PCP) and *Mycobacterium avium* complex (MAC) is warranted.
4. Early diagnosis and treatment of opportunistic infection
   Effective early diagnosis requires a good physician-patient relationship, close patient follow-up, and attention to patient education.
5. Optimizing the quality of life
   Careful attention to psychosocial issues, financial matters, and issues of death and dying is important.

ESSENTIAL PATHOPHYSIOLOGY AND MEDICAL MANAGEMENT OF HIV INFECTION

Human immunodeficiency virus (HIV) attaches to cells at the CD4 receptor. CD4 receptors are found on many cells of the body, including cells of the central nervous system (CNS), GI tract, and immune system (the CD4 or T4 lymphocyte). At the time of HIV infection, the average number of CD4 cells per ml of blood is about 1,000, although the normal number ranges from about 500 to 1,500. As a result of HIV infection, through mechanisms that are not understood fully, there is a concomitant decline in CD4 number and immune function. The rate of decline varies with each individual; an average interval from initial infection to development of AIDS is approximately 10 years.

Medical management of HIV infection consists of:

- Monitoring CD4 count
- Offering antiretroviral therapy when CD4 count falls below 500
- Initiating prophylaxis against PCP at a CD4 count of 200 or less
- Initiating prophylaxis against MAC at a CD4 count of 50 or less

Additionally, the HIV-infected individual must be monitored closely for the development of opportunistic processes (Fig 3–1).

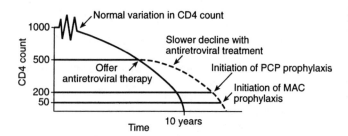

Figure 3–1. CD4 Interpretation.

4

Initial Patient Visit

Report all new AIDS cases to the Centers for Disease Control and Prevention via the local health department (see Appendix for AIDS definition and CDC reporting form).

History

A general history of the patient is critical. Specific questions are indicated regarding mode of infection and possible dates of infection. Occurrence of any HIV-related problems or AIDS-defining illness must be documented. Current medication should be noted, including vitamins or other substances taken for nutritional or medicinal purposes.

Past Medical History

Special attention should be paid to sexually transmitted diseases (including hepatitis, syphilis, venereal warts, herpes) and fungal (ie, coccidioidomycosis and histoplasmosis if in or from an endemic area), parasitic, and mycobacterial infections. Dates and treatment should be noted.

Review of Systems

Is the patient experiencing any of the following?

- Fatigue
- Weight loss, anorexia
- Anxiety, depression
- Fever, chills, night sweats
- Adenopathy
- Skin rash
- Bruises, other skin lesions
- Headache, sinusitis
- Blurring of vision (or other visual changes)
- Oral sores
- Dysphagia or odynophagia
- Shortness of breath or dyspnea on exertion
- Cough
- Abdominal pain
- Nausea, vomiting, diarrhea, constipation
- Rectal sores, genital sores
- Arthritis, muscle weakness
- Forgetfulness
- Lack of coordination

Psychosocial History

Information regarding living conditions of the patient (including prior travel and residence) is important and should be elicited. A genogram with the names of past and present sexual partners, close friends, and relatives can be useful. Notate telephone access, transportation and community resources, psychological and emotional support systems, employment, financial, and medical resources.

Expectations and Questions

Patients should be asked about familiarity and experiences with others having HIV infection. A dialogue regarding individual expectations of immediate and long-term prospects should be initiated and continued throughout treatment. Patients may have strong feelings regarding the level of intervention they desire, particularly in regard to life-prolonging measures (see section of Appendix, "Living Will").

Physical Examination

A complete physical examination is required. Vital signs should include weight and temperature. Careful documentation of the oral, funduscopic, lymphatic, abdominal (liver and spleen), genital (pelvic examination for women), rectal, neurologic, dermatologic and mental status examinations is recommended (see section of Appendix, "Mental Status Examination").

Laboratory

Laboratory tests to be performed on the initial visit include:

1. Hematologic: CBC with differential, platelets, reticulocytes and absolute CD4 count
2. Chemistry: SMAC, serum albumin (vitamins B_{12} and B_6 and zinc levels optional)
3. RPR
4. Hepatitis BsAg and Ab (prior to immunization)
5. Coccidioidomycosis serology (when indicated)
6. Toxoplasmosis serology
7. Chest x-ray, PA (lateral optional)
8. PPD with 2 controls (see section on Tuberculosis for details of PPD and anergy testing)
9. PAP smear for women (see Chapter 10, "HIV Infection in Women").

While P-24 antigen and β_2 microglobulin tests are recommended for HIV-infected persons, at this time they are not used as a basis for clinical decision making and do not need to be drawn routinely.

Health Maintenance

- Immunizations
  Pneumococcal vaccine. Should be given at earliest opportunity following diagnosis of HIV infection.
  Influenza vaccine. Administer yearly.
  MMR. May be given if indicated.
  Td. Update every 10 years or as indicated.
  H influenzae **type b vaccine.** Optional.
  Hepatitis B vaccine. Consider on an individual basis.
- *Haemophilus influenzae* type b vaccine may be offered to patients. Individuals infected with HIV are at increased risk of invasive *H influenzae* infections. Some studies have shown that early in infection, HIV-infected patients are able to mount an antibody response that may confer protection against *H influenzae* type b. However, another study suggests that in HIV-infected persons, most *H influenzae* infections are not type b.
- Consider immune globulin after measles exposure and varicella-zoster immune globulin (VZIg) and hepatitis B immune globulin (HBIg) after exposures.
- Social service assessment of financial, housing, food, and psychologic and emotional needs (with appropriate intervention) is essential.
- Reproductive counseling and contraception should be discussed early on with HIV-infected women of childbearing age (see Chapter 10, "HIV Infection in Women"). Heterosexual and bisexual men also benefit from counseling.
- Nutrition is especially important for HIV-infected individuals. Multivitamin and mineral supplements, at the very least, are recommended for HIV-infected patients (see Chapter 12, "HIV and Nutrition").
- Exercise, risk reduction, and safer sex practices should be discussed. Smoking cessation, injecting-drug use cessation, and exercise have been shown to be beneficial to those infected with HIV. Frank discussions including the use of "clean needles" and safer sexual practices are essential. Further, even after HIV infection, avoiding risky behavior and preventing repeat infection or immune stimulation will contribute to overall health and may prolong life.

- Exploration of community resources should be encouraged. Obtaining printed material from local resources for patients' personal reference is helpful and advised.
- PPD and 2 controls should be repeated yearly unless patient is PPD-positive or has been anergic in 2 prior testings (see section on Tuberculosis for details).

REFERENCES

Centers for Disease Control and Prevention. Recommendations of the Advisory Committee on Immunization Practices (ACIP): Use of vaccine and immune globulins in persons with altered immunocompetence. *MMWR* 1993;**42(No RR-5):**1.

Royce RA, Winkelstein W: HIV infection, cigarette smoking, and CD4+ T-lymphocyte counts: Preliminary results from the San Francisco Men's Health Study. *AIDS* 1990;**4:**327.

Schlenzig C, Jaeger H, Wehrenberg M, et al: Physical exercise favorably influences the course of illness in patients with HIV and AIDS. In: *Program and abstracts of the Eighth International Conference on AIDS/III STD World Congress.* July 19–24, 1992; Amsterdam, the Netherlands. Abstract PoB3401.

Steinhart R et al: Invasive *Haemophilus influenzae* infections in men with HIV infection. *JAMA* 1992;**268:**3350.

Steinhoff MC et al: Antibody response to *Haemophilus influenzae* type b vaccines in men with human immunodeficiency virus infection. *N Engl J Med* 1991;**325:**1837.

Weber R, Ledergerber B, Opravil M et al: Progression of HIV infection in misusers of injected drugs who stop injecting or follow a program of maintenance treatment with methadone. *BMJ* 1990;**301:**1362.

5
Follow-Up Examination

The follow-up visit should be scheduled as soon as possible after lab results have become available—generally within 1–2 weeks.

Interval History

Particular emphasis should be given to the psychosocial dimensions of the patient's response to HIV infection (see Chapter 4, "Initial Patient Visit").

Review of Systems

A review of systems should be performed at each visit.

Physical Examination

A physical examination is indicated at each visit.

Interpretation of Laboratory Results

CBC: Anemia is common and may be a result of direct effect of HIV, marrow infection or malignancy, or medication. Treatable causes must be excluded as with any anemia. Bone marrow biopsy (if indicated) should include studies for: fungi, *Mycobacterium avium* complex (MAC), *Mycobacterium* tuberculosis (MTb), cytomegalovirus (CMV), *Parvovirus,* and malignancy.

Platelets: Thrombocytopenia is seen in HIV infection. Early in infection, it is generally because of idiopathic thrombocytopenic purpura (ITP). Late in infection, it is generally a result of decreased production of platelets secondary to marrow suppression. Thrombocytopenia can also be seen in association with Kaposi's sarcoma.

Differential: Leukopenia is common in HIV infection. White-cell counts of less than 2,000 are common and as a sole indicator are not cause for undue alarm. It is unknown if neutropenia (absolute neutrophil count < 750) increases risk of infection in HIV-infected persons. When using multiple medications that cause neutropenia, colony-stimulating factors such as filgrastim (Neupogen) may be necessary to compensate.

Chemistry: Renal function may be impaired as a result of HIV nephropathy or volume depletion from diarrhea or wasting. Protein and globulin may be elevated as a nonspecific finding. Hepatitis may be due to infection (Hepatitis B virus [HBV], CMV, Hepatitis C, etc) or medications. Elevated LDH may be nonspecific or in response to pulmonary infection, especially *Pneumocystis carinii* pneumonia (PCP). In the absence of infection, elevated LDH may be a result of lymphoma, hemolysis, or muscle wasting caused by HIV or zidovudine. Elevated triglycerides are frequent and are viewed as a response to cytokine activation. Vitamins B_{12}, B_6, and zinc are frequently deficient in HIV-infected patients. Low albumin levels are indicative of malnutrition (see Chapter 12, "HIV and Nutrition").

PPD: In HIV-infected persons, a PPD of 5 mm induration or greater is considered positive. Patients who do not react to either of the controls, nor to the PPD, are likely anergic; chest x-ray is then indicated (see section on Tuberculosis).

CD4 Cells: As HIV infects CD4 cells, the absolute count of CD4 cells (T-helper or T4 cells) is the most clinically useful status indicator of the HIV-infected individuals' immune system. Periodic evaluation of CD4 count is critical in establishing the risk of opportunistic infections and in following the progress of the HIV infection.

For purposes of both long- and short-term evaluation, patients may be divided into 3 groups based on CD4 count.

1: CD4 > 500—Patients are at low risk for AIDS-defining opportunistic infections. They may, however, be at increased risk for tuberculosis, varicella-zoster, recurrent herpes simplex, and bacterial infections (especially *Salmonella, H influenzae,* and *S pneumoniae*). No PCP prophylaxis is indicated. Antiretroviral therapy is controversial in this group. Results of 1 report indicate that disease progression was significantly less frequent in individuals taking zidovudine (median CD4 count was 595).

2: CD4 < 500 but > 200—Patients are at low-to-moderate risk for opportunistic infection. PCP prophylaxis is typically not indicated. Individuals may show some symptoms of HIV infection such as weight loss, diarrhea, lymphadenopathy, and fever. Dermatologic problems, *Candida,* MTb, varicella-zoster, herpes simplex, and Kaposi's sarcoma are more common than in persons with CD4 count > 500.

Zidovudine has been evaluated in patients with CD4 cell count < 500 and has been shown to delay the decline in CD4. Results have been generalized to apply to other antiretroviral medications. Appropriate antiretroviral therapy should be offered to all persons with CD4 count of < 500 (see Chapter 7, "Antiretroviral Therapy").

3: CD4 < 200—Patients have AIDS by CD4 criteria and are at high risk for opportunistic infection.

Antiretroviral therapy is indicated. Prophylaxis for PCP and MAC and other opportunistic infections should be initiated at appropriate times (see Chapter 6, "Prophylaxis Against Opportunistic Infections").

Frequency of Follow-Up

Clinical status determines how often a patient needs follow-up appointments. Additionally, individual psychosocial status will influence frequency of follow-up visits. (Many patients prefer a monthly follow-up.) The CD4 count must be monitored; the frequency necessary for adequate monitoring determines the minimum interval of follow-up required.

A CD4 count for each patient with HIV infection should be obtained every 3–6 months.

Because the CD4 count is currently the single most useful

test for clinical decision-making, it tends to be the focus of much attention by both physicians and infected individuals. It is important to recognize there is considerable variability in CD4 counts. It is advised to focus on broad groupings, as previously described, and to limit the significance of minor fluctuations seen in repeated measurements.

Calculation of Absolute CD4 Count

No. of WBC × %lymphs × %CD4 = Absolute CD4 Count
(eg, 5,000 × .20 × .30 = 300)

REFERENCES

Cooper D et al: Zidovudine in persons with asymptomatic HIV infection and CD4+ cell counts greater than 400 per cubic millimeter. *N Engl J Med* 1993;**329**:297.

6

Prophylaxis Against Opportunistic Infections

Prevention is a key concept in the care of HIV-infected individuals—the prevention of viral transmission, prevention of illness by immunizing patients, and prevention of opportunistic infections. Currently there are numerous clinical trials underway on prophylactic regimens for some of the most common opportunistic infections.

PNEUMOCYSTIS CARINII PNEUMONIA PROPHYLAXIS

Pneumocystis carinii pneumonia (PCP) is the most common opportunistic infection in untreated HIV-infected individuals. Appropriate PCP prophylaxis continues to be the single most important intervention that medicine has to offer the HIV-infected person at this time. Although recommendations in this manual are based on the CDC guidelines, the following medication and dose recommendations are somewhat different than current CDC recommendations; however they are consistent with available research and the practice of other experts. Please see the *Pneumocystis carinii* section for more details on diagnosis and treatment.

Indications for Primary Prophylaxis

- Patients with CD4 < 200
- Patients with AIDS or other signs of immune suppression (ie, oral candidiasis, persistent unexplained fever) regardless of CD4 number.

Indications for Secondary Prophylaxis

Patients with previous PCP.

Medications for Prophylaxis

Trimethoprim/Sulfamethoxazole (Bactrim, Septra): Currently, 1 double strength (DS) tablet 3 times weekly (MWF) for primary and secondary prophylaxis is recommended. The most common side effects are nausea, vomiting, fever, skin rashes—including Stevens-Johnson syndrome, elevated liver function tests, and bone marrow suppression. Patients may be continued on TMP/SMX if the symptoms are mild and these symptoms generally resolve. Desensitization may be effective in selected patients (see "Appendix," section on TMP/SMX Desensitization Protocol). Bone marrow suppression is more common in patients on other marrow suppressive drugs, especially zidovudine or ganciclovir. Although data have not been published, bone marrow suppression may respond to folinic acid (leucovorin) 10–20 mg PO daily. Severe reactions require alternative regimens.

Dapsone: Currently, 100 mg PO QD for primary and secondary prophylaxis is recommended. Side effects include anemia, increased LDH, peripheral neuropathy, methemoglobinemia, nausea, and skin rashes. Dapsone is frequently well tolerated by those intolerant of TMP/SMX. In patients with low glucose-6-phosphate-dehydrogenase (G6PD) levels, hemolysis may occur. Patients who develop anemia while taking dapsone should be evaluated for hemolysis.

Pentamidine: Pentamidine is used intravenously as therapy for acute PCP. It is also used in an aerosolized form for PCP prophylaxis. Currently, the FDA and the manufacturer recommend 300 mg monthly via Respirgard II nebulizer or 60 mg every 2 weeks by Fisoneb ultrasonic hand-held nebulizer (after a loading dose of five 60-mg doses 24–72 hours apart over a 2 week period). Side effects include cough, bronchospasm, metallic taste in the mouth, and sometimes hypoglycemia. As pentamidine has come into widespread use, there have been increasing numbers of cases of extrapulmonary pneumocystosis, recurrent PCP in the upper lobes and pneumothorax. It is believed this recurrent PCP in the upper lobes may be due to poor delivery of drug to the upper lobes.

In order to minimize the risk of tuberculosis transmission to health personnel, excluding tuberculosis (PPD, CXR and sputums as indicated) before commencing pentamidine inhalation is advised.

Choice of Prophylactic Regimen

TMP/SMX is the initial drug of choice for primary and secondary PCP prophylaxis. Dapsone is used if the patients are intolerant of TMP/SMX. Pentamidine is generally reserved for patients intolerant of the other drugs or with severe anemia or granulocytopenia.

MYCOBACTERIUM AVIUM COMPLEX PROPHYLAXIS

Mycobacterium avium complex (MAC) infection is the most common bacterial infection in patients with advanced HIV disease. The incidence of MAC bacteremia increases exponentially as the CD4 count approaches zero with the majority of cases occurring in patients with CD4 counts < 50. The treatment of MAC is difficult at best (see Chapter 8, the section on MAC, for treatment details). There has been considerable interest in prophylaxis against MAC.

Three drugs have been researched or are currently under investigation: clarithromycin, clofazamine, and rifabutin. Clofazamine was investigated by Abrams and found not to be effective in prophylaxis. Rifabutin was investigated in 2 trials conducted by Adria Laboratories. A total of 1146 patients with CD4 < 200 were followed. Approximately 18% of a placebo group versus 9% of the group treated with rifabutin developed MAC bacteremia. Survival was not prolonged, but there was a trend in that direction. Based on this information, the FDA approved rifabutin in late 1992 for the prevention of disseminated MAC in patients with advanced HIV disease. Some experts are concerned about the potential of MAC to develop resistance to single agents used for treatment and prophylaxis. In the case of rifabutin, this also could have implications for tuberculosis treatment where rifampin (a close relative of rifabutin) is a mainstay of treatment. Clarithromycin is active against MAC and is approved for the treatment of MAC in combination with other agents for the treatment of MAC. It is currently under investigation as a potential prophylactic agent, for use alone or in combination with rifabutin.

Before initiating prophylaxis, patients should be evaluated for MAC and tuberculosis.

Indications for MAC Prophylaxis

The following indication for MAC prophylaxis is somewhat different than the current CDC recommendation; however, it is consistent with available research and the practice of other experts.

- Patients with CD4 < 50 and without mycobacterial disease should be considered for MAC prophylaxis.

Medications for Prophylaxis

Rifabutin: At this time, the recommended dose of rifabutin is 300 mg daily (as a single dose or divided BID) for patients with CD4 < 50 who do not have mycobacterial disease.

While rifabutin is generally well tolerated, it may cause rashes, gastrointestinal intolerance, and neutropenia. Uveitis has also been described; symptoms include eye pain, photophobia, erythema, and blurred vision. Rifabutin also has liver enzyme inducing properties and may reduce the activity of other drugs including dapsone, narcotics including methadone, oral contraceptives, anticoagulants, etc. There is also a decrease in plasma levels of zidovudine (however dose changes are not recommended), but no effect on didanosine. Co-administration with clarithromycin may result in increased plasma levels and toxicities. Patients being treated for tuberculosis should not receive rifabutin for MAC prophylaxis. Patients should be warned that there may be some orange discoloration of urine and other body secretions.

Other Medications

Currently rifabutin is the only medication shown to be effective in MAC prophylaxis. Prior to the approval of rifabutin, many clinicians were using clarithromycin or azithromycin in an attempt at prophylaxis. Investigations into other prophylactic regimens are in progress, including the use of clarithromycin alone or in combination with rifabutin.

TOXOPLASMOSIS ENCEPHALITIS PROPHYLAXIS

There is considerable interest in primary prophylaxis against toxoplasmosis encephalitis. Many agents are under investigation including pyrimethamine, dapsone, TMP/SMX, fansidar, and clarithromycin. There is retrospective data that TMP/SMX, when used in doses equivalent to those used for PCP prophylaxis, provides protection against cerebral toxoplasmosis. There is also evidence that pyrimethamine alone *may* increase mortality when used as primary prophylaxis. Pyrimethamine, however, in a French trial was found to be highly effective in preventing toxoplasmosis encephalitis when used in combination with dapsone.

RECOMMENDATION

It is recommended that patients with positive toxoplasmosis serology and < 200 CD4 cells take TMP/SMX (double-strength) 3 times weekly in order to prevent both PCP and toxoplasmosis encephalitis. For those patients unable to tolerate TMP/SMX, dapsone 100 mg PO QD plus pyrimethamine 50 mg per week (with folinic acid 25 mg/week) is recommended.

Secondary prophylaxis, which is really suppressive therapy for those with the disease, is discussed in Chapter 8 in the section discussing *Toxoplasma gondi*.

FUNGAL PROPHYLAXIS

There is some interest in the use of fluconazole as primary prophylaxis for systemic fungal infections (including *Candida, Cryptococcus*, histoplasmosis, coccidioidomycosis) and clinical trials are underway. Recent data were released from a randomized trial comparing fluconazole and clotrimazole troches for the prevention of invasive fungal infections in patients with advanced HIV disease. Fluconazole (200 mg PO daily) significantly delayed both superficial fungal infections and serious mycoses. Survival benefits could not be assessed because of the low incidence of fatalities. Many clinicians are liberal in the use of continuous fluconazole at doses of 100 mg daily or 3 days per week in patients with recurrent oral, vaginal, or esophageal candidiasis. The chronic use of fluconazole has been associated with fluconazole-resistant *Candida*.

Recommendation

At this time, there is not sufficient evidence to support the use of this or any agent as primary prophylaxis against systemic fungal infections. However, in the absence of any data, the use of systemic antifungals in those patients with recurrent candidiasis is advised. Fluconazole is effective and well tolerated. It is also expensive. Secondary prophylaxis of *Cryptococcus noformans* or *Coccidioides immitis* is really suppressive treatment and is discussed in the treatment section of this book.

HERPES SIMPLEX PROPHYLAXIS

As immune system function declines in the face of HIV infection, reactivation of latent Herpes simplex virus (HSV) infection becomes increasingly problematic. There is considerable evidence that acyclovir in doses of 200 mg TID or 400 mg BID is effective in suppressing recurrent outbreaks.

Recommendation

It is recommended that people with recurrent HSV infection receive suppressive acyclovir at 200 mg PO TID or 400 mg PO BID. Clinicians should be aware that acyclovir resistant strains of HSV have been reported, and they should monitor for this occurrence.

CYTOMEGALOVIRUS PROPHYLAXIS

There has been interest in the use of high dose acyclovir to prevent the development of cytomegalovirus (CMV) infection/disease. At this time there are no data supportive of this practice. A prodrug of acyclovir (valacyclovir HCl), which is rapidly converted to acyclovir and results in a 3- or 4-fold increase in acyclovir bioavailability, is under evaluation. In addition, an oral formulation of ganciclovir is currently in clinical trials to determine its prophylactic effectiveness.

Recommendation

At the current time, specific prophylaxis for CMV is not recommended. The treatment of CMV generally requires long-term administration of either ganciclovir or foscarnet. For details, please see the treatment section of this book.

REFERENCES

Abrams DI et al: Clofazamine as prophylaxis for disseminated *Mycobacterium avium* complex infection in AIDS. *J Infect Dis* 1993;**167**:1459.

Blum RN et al: Comparative trial of dapsone versus trimethoprim/sulfamethoxaole for primary prophylaxis of *Pneumocystis carinii* pneumonia. *J Acquir Immune Defic Syndr* 1992;**5**:341.

Carr A et al: Low-dose trimethoprim-sulfasoxazole prophylaxis for toxoplasmic encephalitis in patients with AIDS. *Ann Inter Med* 1992;**117**:106.

Carr A et al: Trimethoprim-sulfamethoxazole appears more effective than aerosolized pentamidine as secondary prophylaxis against *Pneumocystis carinii* pneumonia in patients with AIDS. *AIDS* 1992;**6**:165.

Centers for Disease Control. Recommendations for prophylaxis against *Pneumocystis carinii* pneumonia for adults and adolescents infected with human immunodeficiency virus. *MMWR* 1992;**41(No. RR–4)**:1.

Centers for Disease Control and Prevention. Recommendations for counseling persons infected with human T-lymphotrophic virus, types I and II. Recommendations on prophylaxis and therapy for disseminated *Mycobacterium avium* complex for adults and adolescents infected with human immunodeficiency virus. *MMWR* 1993;**42(No. RR–9)**:17.

Conant MA: Prophylactic and suppressive treatment with acyclovir and the management of herpes in patients with acquired immunodeficiency syndrome. *J Am Acad Derm* 1988;**18**:186.

Feinberg J: Another look at MAC prophylaxis. *AIDS Clinical Care* 1993;**5**:96.

Girard PM et al: Dapsone-pyrimethamine compared with aerosolized pentamidine as primary prophylaxis against *Pneumocystis carinii* pneumonia and toxoplasmosis. *N Engl J Med* 1993;**328**:1514.

Hardy WD et al: A controlled trial of trimethoprim-sulfamethoxazole or aerosolized pentamidine for secondary prophylaxis of *Pneumocystis carinii* pneumonia in patients with the acquired immunodeficiency syndrome. AIDS clinical trials group protocol 021. *N Engl J Med* 1992;**327**:1842.

Letter to physicians from Burroughs Wellcome Co. August 10, 1992.

Jewett JF, Hect FM: Preventive health care for adults with HIV infection. *JAMA* 1993;**269**:1144.

Martin MA et al: A comparison of the effectiveness of 3 regimens in the prevention of carinii pneumonia in human immunodeficiency virus-infected patients. *Arch Intern Med* 1992;**152**:523.

Masur H: Prevention and treatment of pneumocystis pneumonia. *N Engl Med* 1992;**327**:1853.

Newman S et al: Clinically significant *Candida* mucositis resistant to high dose fluconazole in patients with AIDS. IX International Conference on AIDS, Berlin 1993;Abstract PO-B09-1372.

Nightingale S et al: Incidence of *Mycobacterium avium*-intracellulare complex bacteremia in human immunodeficiency virus-positive patients. *J Infect Dis* 1992;**165**:1082.

Nightingale SD et al: Two controlled trials of rifabutin prophylaxis against *Mycobacterium avium* complex infection in AIDS. *New Engl J Med* 1993;**329**:823.

Nightingale SD et al: Primary prophylaxis with fluconazole against systemic fungal infections in HIV-positive patients. *AIDS* 1992;**6**:191.

Ruskin J, LaRiviere M: Low dose co-trimoxazole for prevention of *Pneumocystis carinii* pneumonia in human immunodeficiency virus disease. *Lancet* 1991;**337**:468.

Sanguineti A, Carmichael JK, Campbell K: Fluconazole-resistant *Candida albicans* after long-term suppression therapy. *Arch Intern Med* 1993;**153**:1122.

Schneider MME et al: A controlled trial of aerosolized pentamidine of trimethoprim-sulfamethoxasole as primary prophylaxis against *Pneumocystis carinii* pneumonia in patients with human immunodeficiency virus infection. *N Engl J Med* 1992;**327**:1836.

Sepkowitz KA et al: Pneumothorax in AIDS. *Ann Int Med* 1991;**114**:455.

7

Antiretroviral Therapy & Strategy

ANTIRETROVIRAL AGENTS

At this time, there are four antiretroviral medications available to physicians, zidovudine, didanosine, zalcitabine, and stavudine. All are reverse transcriptase inhibitors. Considerable research has been completed regarding optimal antiretroviral therapy; however, much research is still in progress and many issues remain to be clarified.

There are 3 major considerations in the evaluation of antiretroviral therapy:

1. The toxicity of the medications
2. The duration of effectiveness of the currently available drugs, especially in advanced disease
3. Reverse transcriptase inhibitors do not completely suppress viral replication. This allows for continued destruction of the immune system despite antiretroviral therapy

In this section each of the available antiretroviral medications will be reviewed. In the following section, an antiretroviral strategy consistent with the currently available data will be suggested.

Zidovudine (ZDV, formerly AZT; Trade name–Retrovir)

Indications: Zidovudine is indicated for people with HIV infection who have a CD4 count < 500.

Discussion of Indications: Multiple investigations have shown that asymptomatic patients with absolute CD4 counts of < 500, benefit from taking zidovudine, which results in slower decline in CD4 counts and longer time to development of opportunistic infection. However, zidovudine has not been demonstrated to prolong long-term survival.

Zidovudine is indicated for symptomatic HIV disease and is superior to didanosine and zalcitabine as first line therapy. Zidovudine is currently the initial drug of choice.

While there is still some controversy regarding the optimal time of initiation, offering asymptomatic patients the option of initiating zidovudine when the CD4 count is < 500 is recommended.

Patients with > 500 CD4 cells may also benefit from zidovudine. Research in this area is ongoing. It is known that zidovudine and other nucleosides lose effectiveness over time, especially in advanced HIV disease. The reasons for this are not fully understood, but appear to relate to incomplete suppression of viral replication, development of drug resistance, decreased drug phosphorylation, and the development of syncytium-inducing (SI) viral phenotypes. There are increasing data that show worse clinical outcome among patients with highly resistant virus.

Dosage: The optimal dose of zidovudine is 500–600 mg/day. A recent report suggested 300 mg/day had clinical and virologic activity but was not necessarily optimal. Another study investigating combination therapy found that 150 mg/day was not effective.

A dose of 200 mg PO TID is recommended. Patients who are intolerant of this dose may tolerate lower doses. The minimal active dose seems to be 100 mg PO TID; this is acceptable, although not optimal.

Toxicity and Side Effects: The primary toxicity of zidovudine is hematologic. Patients tolerant of zidovudine generally develop a mild macrocytosis with or without anemia within 2 months. This is not a reason to stop zidovudine. Normocytic anemia may develop and is of greater concern because it may precede severe anemia. In cases of severe anemia, zidovudine should be reduced or discontinued, and transfusions given as needed. Severe persistent anemia may respond to erythropoietin. Other causes of anemia, particularly infections, need to be considered. Patients with persistent or severe recurrent anemia should be considered for alternate antiretroviral therapy such as didanosine or zalcitabine.

Neutropenia is a major side effect that limits therapy. Recent studies indicate that zidovudine may be continued safely until the absolute neutrophil count (ANC) declines to < 750 (ANC = No. WBC × % neutrophils). Growth stimulating factors (ie, filgrastim) may be considered but alternative therapy with didanosine or zalcitabine may be preferable.

Headache, insomnia, and gastrointestinal symptoms are often seen early after beginning zidovudine. They generally resolve in a few weeks with symptomatic treatment. Occasionally these toxicities will require discontinuation of zidovudine. Some clinicians initiate therapy at 1 capsule daily and increase the dose by 1 capsule every 2–3 days until the target dose is reached. This appears to decrease some of the headache and GI distress associated with the initiation of zidovudine. Administering zidovudine with meals may also minimize such complaints.

Myopathy or myositis may be seen after long-term use of zidovudine (generally more than 1 year). Myalgias, muscle wasting, and weakness as well as increased CPK are seen and may require dose reduction or interruption.

Steatosis with hepatomegaly and elevated liver function tests may be drug related and require drug discontinuation. Nail pigmentation may also be noted.

Contrary to earlier thinking, acetaminophen is not contraindicated with zidovudine.

Rifabutin and clarithromycin lower plasma zidovudine levels but no dose adjustment is recommended at this time.

Monitoring: Initial laboratory tests include a CBC with differential and platelets. Repeat the CBC and differential at 2 weeks, 1, 2, and 3 months and then every 3 months unless there are indications of intolerance. If there are indications of intolerance, follow-up as clinically indicated.

Didanosine (ddI; Trade name–Videx)

Indications: Didanosine has been approved by the FDA for the following indications:

1. Patients over 6 months of age who are intolerant of zidovudine
2. Patients with "clinical or immunologic deterioration" during zidovudine therapy
3. Patients who have received prior prolonged zidovudine therapy.

Discussion of indications:

1. Patients over 6 months who are intolerant of zidovudine.

    Patients who do not tolerate zidovudine should be offered therapy with didanosine.

2. Patients who have demonstrated "clinical or immunologic deterioration" during zidovudine therapy.

    "Clinical or immunologic deterioration" has not been defined by the FDA. A recently published definition based on CD4 number appears reasonable:

- For people who began zidovudine with 250–500 CD4 cells; either a 50% decline in counts or a decline to < 200 on 2 occasions separated by at least 4 weeks.
- For those with 100–250 CD4 cells; a 50% decrease in counts or a decline to < 50 on 2 occasions separated by at least 4 weeks.
- Clinicians may want to take into account the duration of zidovudine therapy in people meeting these criteria as some experts believe that patients who have received zidovudine for only a short time may continue to benefit from zidovudine despite falling CD4 counts.

3. Patients who have received prior prolonged zidovudine therapy.

   This new indication is based on the findings of the ACTG study 116B/117. This study showed that patients who had been on zidovudine for a median of 13.7 months (range 3–61 months) and changed to didanosine had significantly fewer AIDS defining events and deaths than those who were continued on zidovudine.

Dosage: Please note new doses based on ACTG study 116B/117.

Adult Dosing–

Patient Weight	Tablets
≥ 60 kg	200 mg PO BID
< 60 kg– 45 kg	125 mg PO BID
< 45 kg	100 mg PO BID

Note: Each dose of the tablet formulation must include 2 tablets in order to provide adequate buffer, thus 200 mg PO BID is really two 100 mg tabs PO BID. Didanosine should be taken on an empty stomach.

Tablets must be thoroughly chewed or crushed and followed by a glass of cold water, or they may be dispersed in cold water and swallowed.

When drug absorption is affected by the level of acidity in the stomach, notably dapsone or ketoconazole, these medications should be taken at least 2 hours after didanosine.

Quinolone antibiotics should not be taken within 2 hours of didanosine.

Tetracyclines should not be taken with didanosine because of the aluminum and magnesium buffer.

Patients with renal impairment or hepatic impairment may require decreased dosages.

Toxicity and Side Effects: The major toxicities of didanosine include hyperamylasemia, pancreatitis and peripheral neuropathy.

- Pancreatitis was seen in about 10% of patients taking didanosine at or below the recommended dosage. In some instances, the disease was fulminant and fatal. Patients with a history of pancreatitis or significant risk factors (alcohol consumption or elevated triglycerides), must be followed closely. Many clinicians will not prescribe didanosine for patients with a recent history of pancreatitis.
- Hyperamylasemia was seen in about 18% of patients taking didanosine and is associated with an increased risk for pancreatitis.
- Peripheral neuropathy has occurred in patients taking didanosine at or below the recommended dosage. Patients should be monitored for the development of a neuropathy that is characterized by distal numbness, tingling, or pain in the feet or hands.

Monitoring: The manufacturer makes no recommendations for monitoring. During the expanded access program a physical examination, chemistry panel, amylase, and CPK were required on a monthly basis.

It is recommended that clinicians follow patients at 2 weeks and then monthly with a physical examination (ask about abdominal pain and neuropathy symptoms) and a chemistry panel with amylase. Physicians should also warn patients to report any abdominal pain immediately. If patients are doing well after 3–6 months, the follow-up may be less frequent.

Zalcitabine (ddC; Trade name–Hivid)

Indications: The FDA has approved zalcitabine to be used in combination with zidovudine for the treatment of adult patients with advanced HIV infection (CD4 < 300) who have demonstrated clinical or immunologic deterioration. Zalcitabine is also indicated as monotherapy for those who have failed or are intolerant of zidovudine.

Discussion of Indications: Zalcitabine was initially FDA-approved only for use in combination with zidovudine for the treatment of adult patients with advanced HIV infection (CD4 < 300) who had demonstrated clinical or immunologic deterioration.

The ACTG 114 trial, which compared zidovudine with zalcitabine as first line therapy in patients with < 200 CD4 cells, was terminated after interim analysis revealed zidovudine superior in terms of prolonging life.

The CPCRA 002 trial compared didanosine with zalcitabine for individuals no longer tolerant of (or failing) zidovudine. Zalcitabine was found to be at least as effective as didanosine in delaying disease progression and superior to didanosine in delaying death. The results from this study suggest that zalcitabine may be an acceptable alternative monotherapy to didanosine for patients intolerant of (or failing) zidovudine.

Dosage: The recommended dose is 0.750 mg of zalcitabine PO TID. There is no need to reduce the dose of zalcitabine unless the patient weighs < 30 kg.

Toxicity and Side Effects: Toxicities associated with zalcitabine include maculopapular cutaneous eruptions, oral ulcers, fever, pancreatitis, and a painful sensory peripheral neuropathy.

Monitoring: Periodic CBC and SMAC is indicated. Amylase should be followed in those patients at risk for pancreatitis.

Careful monitoring for signs suggestive of peripheral neuropathy is recommended. Zalcitabine should be discontinued if patients develop symptoms of peripheral neuropathy, especially if these symptoms are bilateral and progress for > 72 hours. If symptoms improve to mild levels, zalcitabine may be reintroduced at half the original dose.

Stavudine (D4T; Trade name–Zerit)

Indications: Stavudine was approved in July of 1994 for the treatment of adults with advanced HIV infection who are intolerant of approved therapies with proven clinical benefit or who have experienced significant clinical or immunologic deterioration while receiving other therapies or for whom such therapies are contraindicated.

Discussion of Indications: The approval of stavudine was based on an interim analysis, at 12 weeks, of a phase 3 trial of stavudine versus continued zivodudine in adults with CD4 between 50 and 500 and at least 24 weeks of prior zidovudine.

This interim analysis revealed a mean CD4 increase of 22 cells in those on stavudine versus a mean decrease of 22 cells in those who continued on zidovudine.

Stavudine has also been used in about 10,000 individuals in a parallel track program. This program evaluated two different doses of stavudine, 20 or 40 mg BID in patients > 60 kg and 15 or 30 mg in patients < 60 kg. Interim analysis showed similar survival for each dose group.

Dosage: Dose is based on body weight. Stavudine can be taken with or without food.

Patient Weight	Tablets
> 60 kg	40 mg BID
< 60 kg	30 mg BID

Dose must be adjusted in patients with impaired renal function, and may also be lowered in response to elevated transaminases or in cases of neuropathy.

Toxicity and Side Effects: The most common toxisity associated with stavudine is peripheral neuropathy. Neuropathy occurred in about 15% to 20% of patients in clinical trials. The manufacturer recommends stavudine be discontinued if numbness, tingling, or pain develops in the hands or feet. If symptoms resolve, the drug may be resumed at half the original dose.

Pancreatitis was observed in 1% of patients and was associated with some deaths. Modest elevations in serum transaminases were also observed.

Monitoring: Laboratory monitoring of hepatic and pancreatic function is indicated as well as close clinical follow-up for signs or symptoms of peripheral neuropathy.

REFERENCES

Browne MJ et al: d4T in patients with AIDS or AIDS-related complex: A phase I trial. *J Infect Dis* 1993;**167**:21.

Collier AC et al: A pilot study of low-dose zidovudine in human immunodeficiency virus infection. *N Engl J Med* 1990;**323**:1015.

Cocorde Coordinating Committee: Concorde:MRC/ANRS randomized double-blind controlled trial of immediate and deferred zidovudine in symptom-free HIV infection. *Lancet* 1994;343:87.

Cooper DA et al: Zidovudine in persons with asymptomatic HIV infection and CD4+ cell counts greater than 400 per cubic millimeter. *N Engl J Med* 1993;**329:**297.

ddC Information Amendment January 13, 1992.

Hamilton JD et al: A controlled trial of early versus late treatment with zidovudine in symptomatic human immunodeficiency virus infection: Results of the Veterans Affairs Cooperative Study. *N Engl J Med* 1992;**326:**437.

Kahn J: Clinical issues in using didanosine. *AIDS Clinical Care* 1991;**3:**90.

Kahn JO et al: A controlled trial comparing zidovudine with didanosine in human immunodeficiency virus infection. *N Engl J Med* 1992;**327:**581.

Lange JMA: A placebo-controlled clinical trial of zidovudine in asymptomatic HIV-infected individuals. Presented at third European Conference on the Clinical Aspects of HIV Infection; March 12–13, 1992; Paris, France.

Meng TC et al: Combination therapy with zidovudine and dideoxycytidine in patients with advanced human immunodeficiency virus infection. *Ann Int Med* 1992;**116:**13.

Note to Physicians from the NIH/NIAID February 1, 1993.

Volberding PA et al: Zidovudine in asymptomatic human immunodeficiency virus infection: A controlled trial in persons with fewer than 500 CD4 positive cells per cubic millimeter. *N Engl J Med* 1990;**322:**941.

ANTIRETROVIRAL STRATEGY

There are considerable data regarding antiretroviral therapy, but questions about optimal usage of antiretroviral agents remain. Because of the uncertainties (both scientific and political) surrounding antiretrovirals, it is important to involve the patient in the decision making process.

The National Institute of Allergy and Infectious Diseases (NIAID) recently published recommendations from a state-of-the-art conference on antiretroviral therapy in HIV-infected adults. This section outlines an antiretroviral strategy consistent with the current data and generally consistent with the NIAID recommendations.

Antiretroviral strategy can be divided into 4 sections: (1) antiretroviral naive patients, (2) antiretroviral failure, (3) antiretroviral sequence, and (4) discontinuation of antiretroviral therapy.

Antiretroviral Naive Patients

For patients who have never taken any antiretroviral agent, the initial drug of choice is zidovudine. Zidovudine may be offered when the CD4 count falls below 500.

- CD4 < 500: Zidovudine as monotherapy.

Antiretroviral Failure

Eventually, HIV becomes resistant to current antiretroviral therapy. It appears that resistance develops faster at lower CD4 counts. The decision regarding when to change antiretroviral therapy can be difficult. In selected patients, changing from zidovudine to either didanosine or zalcitabine has been shown to be beneficial. Two combinations commonly used are zidovudine with didanosine and zidovudine with zalcitabine. Didanosine and zalcitabine should not be used together because of similar toxicities.

Until better markers for drug failure exist, a rational approach for altering antiretroviral therapy based on the existing data is not possible. However, some indicators for a change in antiretroviral regimen include:

- Presence of drug toxicity or side effects
- Evidence of disease progression (eg, worsening of HIV-related symptoms or development of new opportunistic infections)
- Declines in CD4 cell counts—for those with CD4 > 200, either a 50% decline or a decline to < 200. For

those with CD4 < 200, a 50% decline or a decline below 50 CD4 cells

Regarding zidovudine therapy, there are data that decreasing effectiveness can be noted after 6–12 months of therapy for those with CD4 cell counts < 100. Until better markers for drug failure or decreasing efficacy are available, changing therapy after approximately 12 months of zidovudine has been suggested.

Antiretroviral Sequence

Anticipation of antiretroviral failure, antiretroviral intolerance, or antiretroviral failure all necessitate change to another regimen. The general sequence of the antiretroviral regimen will be:

- Zidovudine monotherapy *to*
- Didanosine, zalcitabine, or stavudine *or*
- Combination therapy *or*
- Research protocol

In cases of intolerance or patient specific contraindications, it is advisable to try to avoid another drug with the same toxicity. An alternative to changing to another drug might be a brief drug holiday and then a re-trial at a lower dose. If this fails, a closely followed trial of a drug with a similar toxicity may be worthwhile.

Discontinuation of Antiretroviral Therapy

Antiretroviral naive individuals with low CD4 counts show survival benefits when zidovudine is initiated. However, for patients with a history of antiretroviral use, as CD4 counts decline below 50, the relative benefits of continued antiretroviral therapy also decline. Additionally, the frequency of side effects and drug interactions are increased. It may be useful to discontinue antiretroviral therapy late in HIV infection (CD4 < 50), especially in patients with severe side effects or who are on many other medications. This decision must be tailored to each individual and should be made after a detailed discussion with the patient.

REFERENCES

Sande MA et al: Antiretroviral therapy for adult HIV-infected persons. *JAMA* 1993;**270:**2583.

8
Common HIV-Associated Infections & Conditions

CANDIDIASIS

Candida is a fungus that is frequently the first opportunistic infection acquired by HIV-infected people. *Candida* infections are most common in the oral cavity (thrush) and the esophagus. Vaginal, rectal, and cutaneous lesions are also seen.

Presentation

Symptoms: Oral Candida–Despite the presence of oral lesions, patients are often asymptomatic during early stages of the disease. Some patients complain of oral discomfort, a burning sensation when eating, or an altered sense of taste.

Esophageal Candida–Typically presents as odynophagia or dysphagia. Many patients complain of anterior chest pain exacerbated by swallowing.

Physical Findings: Oral Candida–Commonly seen as whitish furry or cheesy exudates on the buccal mucosa, gingiva, tongue, or palate. There may be an erythematous base noted after scraping the lesion. Occasionally the typical white exudate is absent and the only finding is an inflamed or atrophic oral mucosa.

Esophageal Candida–The diagnosis is generally made by history or at endoscopy. Oral thrush may or may not be present concomitant with esophageal candida infection. Esophageal candida may occur in patients taking local therapy (ie, clotrimazole troches).

Diagnosis

Oral Candida–Diagnosis is made by scraping the lesion and examining the collected material under a microscope using KOH preparation. Mycelia will be evident.

Esophageal Candida–A presumptive diagnosis may be made in patients with odynophagia that responds to empiric treatment. Barium swallow may reveal esophageal ulcerations suggestive of *Candida* but it is not diagnostic. Definitive diagnosis is made by endoscopy with biopsy and pathologic or cytologic evidence of *Candida*.

Treatment

Oral Candida–Several therapies are available for oral candidiasis; clotrimazole troches and nystatin swish and swallow are commonly recommended topical therapies. Systemic therapy with ketoconazole, fluconazole, or itraconazole is also available. Ketoconazole at 200 mg MWF provides the least expensive therapy at this time. Many clinicians are quick to institute therapy with fluconazole hoping that there may be some additional prophylactic effect against other fungal infections (fluconazole 100 mg MWF is commonly used).

Esophageal Candida–For most patients with odynophagia or dysphagia, empiric treatment is recommended. The treatment for esophageal candida is fluconazole 100–200 mg PO QD or ketoconazole 200 mg PO BID for 14–21 days. Resolution of symptoms in 2–3 days suggests candida esophagitis. Patients who have had esophageal candida may relapse after treatment and may require continuous systemic low dose prophylaxis as previously described.

Ketoconazole requires an acid pH in the stomach in order for absorption to occur. It is thus recommended to avoid antacids, H2 blockers, or drugs that contain buffering agents such as didanosine, while using ketoconazole.

Candida species resistant to ketoconazole and fluconazole have been reported. Amphotericin is required for treatment of resistant strains.

Itraconazole is a new oral azole with activity against *Candida*. Its role in the treatment of *Candida* is not yet clear.

Other *Candida* Infections

Recurrent and severe vaginal candidiasis is increasingly recognized in HIV-infected women. Although topical treatment is preferred, oral therapy with fluconazole or ketoconazole may be required. Symptomatic rectal candida is often overlooked and undertreated.

COCCIDIOIDOMYCOSIS

Coccidioidomycosis is a fungal disease caused by *Coccidioides immitis* and is endemic in the Southwestern United States, northern Mexico, and parts of Central and South America. In immunocompetent people, most infections are subclinical. However, in immunocompromised people, the disease may be fulminant. Coccidioidomycosis has a variety of presentations and should be considered in the differential of HIV-infected patients with a history of residence or travel in endemic areas.

Presentation

Symptoms: Fish et al identified 6 clinical categories of coccidioidomycosis manifestations in HIV-infected patients:

1. Focal pulmonary
2. Diffuse pulmonary
3. Skin involvement only
4. Meningitis
5. Lymph node or liver
6. Positive serology only

Most patients present with some form of pulmonary coccidioidomycosis. In those patients with relatively high CD4 counts (> 200), it is most likely to occur as a focal pulmonary infiltrate associated with fever, cough, and pleuritic chest pain. This may be hard to distinguish from acute bacterial pneumonia. Those with lower CD4 counts (< 200) generally present with a more severe form, which presents with fever, inanition, and dyspnea associated with a bilateral, diffuse, nodular infiltrate. This may mimic *Pneumocystis carinii* pneumonia. Extrapulmonary disease is less common than the pulmonary forms. Meningitis presents with headache, decreased mentation, and fever. Skin lesions are generally chronic and verrucous in appearance.

Physical Findings: The physical findings are dependent on the organ system involved. Lymphadenopathy is seen occasionally. The coccidioidomycosis skin lesion is variable in appearance, ie, papules, pustules, nodules, ulcers, or large warty lesions as possible manifestations.

Diagnosis

Skin tests for coccidioidomycosis are unreliable in HIV-infected patients and serology is preferred to document exposure.

Mycologic diagnosis is possible through culture of serum, CSF, and biopsy material or other specimens. Cytologic preparations with spherule visualization are of value and often faster than culture.

Serology is useful in diagnosis. IgM and IgG tests are available for both serum and CSF. IgM antibodies occur early in infection and disappear by about 4 months. These antibodies are measured by the "tube precipitin" (TP) method or may be reported directly. Unfortunately, the IgM response is frequently blunted and may be falsely negative in HIV-infected patients. IgG antibodies measured by complement fixation (CF) appear later in infection and are positive in up to 70% of HIV-infected people. CF titers are useful in establishing dissemination with a titer of 1:32 or greater significantly associated with disseminated disease. Titers are also helpful in following response to therapy and in monitoring for breakthrough in patients on suppressive therapy. Titers, however, may not be unreliable in patients with severe immunosuppression.

It is recommended that HIV-infected patients with coccidioidomycosis and headache or other neurologic symptoms undergo a lumbar puncture to exclude meningitis.

Treatment

The definitive therapy for coccidioidomycosis in HIV-infected patients is unknown. It should be appreciated that coccidioidomycosis is a serious disease in immunocompromised persons and that aggressive therapy is generally indicated. Amphotericin B, fluconazole, and itraconazole have been used in the treatment of coccidioidomycosis with some success.

Patients without meningitis should receive amphotericin B at 0.5–1.0 mg/kg daily. If the patient improves over the first few weeks, the dose frequency is changed to 50 mg 3 times weekly until a total dose of 1.0–2.0 grams is reached. After this, long-term suppressant therapy with fluconazole 400 mg daily may be given, but relapses have occurred. Clinically stable patients with either focal pulmonary involvement or disseminated disease without pulmonary involvement may be considered for oral azole therapy for initial and continued suppressive treatment. Antibody titers should be followed to monitor response to therapy and the effectiveness of suppression.

Patients with meningitis are more difficult to treat. Intrathecal amphotericin B has been the standard therapy but recently the good CNS penetration of fluconazole has been encouraging. Coccidioidomycosis meningitis is a serious disease whose definitive treatment is still in evolution. Therefore, consultation with specialists is indicated.

REFERENCES

Ampel NM, Dols CL, Galgiani JN: Coccidioidomycosis during human immunodeficiency virus infection. *Am J Med* 1993;**94:**384.

Bronnimann DA et al: Coccidioidomycosis in the acquired immunodeficiency syndrome. *Ann Int Med* 1987;**106:**372.

Einsten HE, Johnson RH: Coccidioidomycosis: New aspects of epidemiology and therapy. *Clin Inf Dis* 1993;**16:**349.

Fish DG et al: Coccidioidomycosis during human immunodeficiency virus infection. *Medicine* 1990;**69:**384.

Galgiani JN: Coccidioidomycosis. *West J Med* 1993;**159:**153.

Galgiani JN et al: Fluconazole therapy for coccidioidal meningitis. *Ann Int Med* 1993;**119:**28.

CRYPTOCOCCUS NEOFORMANS

Cryptococcus neoformans is a ubiquitous fungus that is found in soil. In normal hosts, after being aerosolized and inhaled, the fungus is contained in the lungs. In immunosuppressed people, the fungus can cause disseminated infection. It accounts for about 5–8% of all opportunistic infections in AIDS. Cryptococcus can cause pulmonary, CNS, or disseminated infection. In people with AIDS, the most common presentation is meningitis. Cryptococcal infections may be fatal if untreated.

Presentation

Symptoms: Onset is insidious with fever, nonspecific fatigue, nausea, and vomiting. Headache may be diffuse, frontal, or temporal. Encephalitis may occur with altered mental status, subtle behavioral changes, memory loss, and confusion. Photophobia, cranial nerve palsies, pneumonia, and painless skin lesions may occur. Prostatic abscesses may serve as a reservoir for recurrent infections.

Physical findings: Meningismus is rare. Papilledema may occur.

Diagnosis

Serum cryptococcal antigen: This test is very sensitive. It may be appropriate to use this test in the evaluation of patients with headache or fever. Some individuals argue that given a positive cryptococcal antigen in serum or urine, treatment should begin based on a diagnosis of disseminated cryptococcus. However, a lumbar puncture should be performed to evaluate for CNS disease. Brain CT or MRI may show the occasional focal granulomas associated with *Cryptococcus* (cryptococcomas).

Lumbar Puncture: Opening pressure, cell count, glucose, and protein should be measured and are often normal in people with HIV-infection and cryptococcal meningitis. Diagnosis can be made by:

1. Positive India ink preparation for fungi
2. Positive CSF cryptococcal antigen (found in 95% of culture-proven CSF)
3. Positive fungal culture.

Treatment

Amphotericin B 0.5–1.0 mg/kg/day IV with or without flucytosine (5FU) 100 mg/kg/day IV divided Q 6 hours until the patient begins to improve or stabilize (2–3 weeks).

Follow with fluconazole 400 mg PO per day for a total of 8–12 weeks.

Once initial treatment is completed, life-long suppressive therapy with fluconazole 200 mg PO daily is recommended.

It is believed that there are some patients who, once disease is diagnosed, may be treated initially with oral fluconazole rather than IV amphotericin. These patients generally have earlier disease and milder symptoms. Specifically, a multicenter study found that patients with a normal mental status, a low CSF cryptococcal titer (< 1:1024), and a CSF WBC count > 20 cells/µg responded equally well to either fluconazole or amphotericin; thus, one could consider using fluconazole as initial therapy. This treatment is still controversial and consultation with knowledgeable specialists is advised. Initial treatment with fluconazole consists of 400 mg QD for 12 weeks.

Patients with increased intracranial pressure tend to have poorer outcomes. Elevated opening pressure readings may be managed with frequent lumbar punctures, mannitol, or corticosteroids.

Both liposomal amphotericin and itraconazole for treatment of cryptococcosis are in clinical trials.

REFERENCES

Feinberg J: Fluconazole vs. amphotericin B for acute cryptococcal meningitis: The pendulum swings back. *AIDS Clinial Care* 1993;**5**:39.

Powderly WG et al: A controlled trial of fluconazole or amphotericin B to prevent relapse of cryptococcal meningitis in patients with the acquired immunodeficiency syndrome. *N Engl J Med* 1992;**326**:793.

Saag MS et al: Comparison of amphotericin B with fluconazole in the treatment of acute cryptococcal meningitis. *N Engl J Med* 1992;**326**:83.

CRYPTOSPORIDIUM, ISOSPORA BELLI, AND *MICROSPORIDA*

The causes of diarrhea and abdominal pain in HIV-infected patients are numerous as illustrated in the list below:

Parasitic: *Cryptosporidium, Isospora belli, Microsporidia, Giardia, Entamoeba histolytica*
Viral: CMV, HSV, adenovirus, enterovirus
Fungal: Candidiasis, histoplasmosis
Bacterial: *MAC, Salmonella, Shigella, Campylobacter, C. difficile*
Neoplasm: Kaposi's sarcoma, lymphoma

The diagnosis and treatment of most of these etiologies is discussed in other sections of this text under the specific organism. The 3 organisms discussed in this chapter are common only to HIV-infected individuals.

Cryptosporidium is a protozoan that causes intractable diarrhea and malabsorption leading to weight loss and malnutrition. Biliary tract obstruction has also been reported. Symptoms may spontaneously improve and worsen.

Isospora belli causes similar symptoms as *Cryptosporidium*. It is more common in tropical and subtropical climates and, thus, is most commonly found in people from these areas.

Microsporida is a small protozoan. The role of *Microsporida* is still unclear because it is difficult to diagnose; thus, its true incidence and symptom complex are unknown. Diagnosis is best made by electron microscopy of small bowel biopsies, although there is beginning to be some success with detecting spores in stool by light microscopy.

Presentation

Please see the discussion of the evaluation of diarrhea in Chpater 9 of this book.

Treatment

Cryptosporidium: *Cryptosporidium* is difficult to treat. Clinical trials are in progress with a few agents. A trial therapy with paromomycin 500 mg PO QID for up to 30 days, with supportive measures such as aggressive antidiarrheal drugs and fluids is suggested. Azithromycin is available from Pfizer on a compassionate basis for the treatment of *Cryptosporidium* (800-742-3029); however, a European study found it to be ineffective. Octreotide may be effective.

Isospora belli: TMP/SMX 160/800 mg PO QID for 10 days followed by TMP/SMX 160/800 mg PO BID for 21 days appears to be effective. Relapse may occur and maintenance therapy may be indicated. Pyrimethamine 75 mg PO

QD plus folinic acid 10–25 mg PO QD is effective in sulfa allergy.

Microsporidia: No effective therapy is known. Metronidazole 500 mg PO TID or albendazole 400 mg PO BID may be beneficial. Antidiarrheal drugs may provide symptomatic relief.

REFERENCES

Armitage K et al: Treatment of *Cryptosporidium* with paromomycin. *Arch Intern Med* 1992;**152:**2497.

Marshall RJ, Flanigan TP: Paromomycin inhibits *Cryptosporidium* infection of a human enterocyte cell line. *J Infect Dis* 1992;**165:**772.

Rabeneck L et al: The role of *Microsporida* in the pathogenesis of HIV-related chronic diarrhea. *Ann Int Med* 1993;**119:**895.

Smith PD et al: Gastrointestinal infections in AIDS. *Ann Int Med* 1992;**116:**63.

Third European Conference on AIDS. Abstract No.P28. Paris, 1992.

Weber et al: Improved light-microscopical detection of *Microsporida spores* in stool and duodenal aspirates. *N Engl J Med* 1992;**326:**161.

Wittner M, Tanowitz HB, Weiss LM: Parasitic infections in AIDS patients. *Infect Dis Clin North Am* 1993;**7:**569.

CYTOMEGALOVIRUS

Cytomegalovirus (CMV) is an important pathogen in HIV-infected people. CMV infection in immunocompetent individuals may provoke a self-limited mono-like illness. In immunocompromised people, CMV may cause chorioretinitis, gastrointestinal disease (colitis, gastritis, esophagitis, proctitis, pancreatitis, and hepatitis), or pneumonia. There also have been reports of CNS and adrenal disease although the frequency and significance of these conditions are unclear. Most patients who develop clinical CMV disease have CD4 counts < 50.

Presentation

Symptoms: Chorioretinitis–Unilateral visual field loss, blurring of vision, or scotomata are the most common symptoms of chorioretinitis. It is important to ask the patient about visual changes at each visit, and promptly refer for ophthalmologic evaluation if a problem is presented.

GI Disease–Generally, colitis is associated with abdominal pain and diarrhea (often hemitest positive). Fever may also be present. Esophagitis and gastritis most commonly present with pain from the involved structures.

Pneumonia–While CMV may be isolated from pulmonary secretions, it is generally believed that it rarely has a true pathologic role in HIV-infected patients. Diagnosis must be confirmed by lung biospy demonstrating histologic evidence consistent with invasive disease.

Physical Findings: Chorioretinitis–Funduscopic examination generally reveals whitish areas with perivascular exudates and hemorrhages. A careful search of the entire fundus is required; thus, ophthalmologic evaluation is recommended.

GI Disease–Endoscopy reveals erythema, submucosal hemorrhage, and diffuse mucosal ulceration.

Pneumonia–Findings are minimal on physical examination.

Neurologic Disease–Encephalitis, cranial nerve dysfunction, or neuropathies may occur. CMV polyradiculopathy is rare, but characterized by lower extremity weakness, numbness, and bladder dysfunction.

Diagnosis

Chorioretinitis: The diagnosis is made solely on the basis of the funduscopic examination. Urine and blood cultures are not useful and they are expensive.

GI Disease: Culture of the virus from tissue obtained during endoscopy is optimal. Histologic examination is important and will reveal characteristic inclusion bodies. There also are fluorescent antibody stains for CMV antigen that may be done on these specimens.

Pneumonia: CXR generally reveals diffuse interstitial infiltrates. Arterial blood gas (ABG) is abnormal with hypoxia and increased alveolar-arterial gradient. Diagnosis is based on positive culture from biopsy, the presence of histologic changes consistent with CMV, and the absence of any other pathogen.

Neurologic Disease: CMV may be isolated from CSF in polyradiculopathy.

Treatment

Ganciclovir and foscarnet are 2 antiviral agents available for the treatment of CMV. Investigations into the use of other drugs are in progress.

Ganciclovir (DHPG): Ganciclovir is effective against CMV and is approved for use in retinitis. Currently, studies are in progress for use in other CMV infections. At this time, ganciclovir is an IV medication. However, an oral formulation is under investigation.

The dose of ganciclovir for CMV retinitis is 5 mg/kg Q 12 hours IV for 14–21 days (induction) followed by 6 mg/kg QD 5–7 days a week for life (maintenance). The dose must be adjusted in patients with renal disease.

Ganciclovir is toxic to the bone marrow and causes neutropenia and anemia. Close follow-up is indicated for patients taking this drug.

Treatment with ganciclovir will arrest the progress of CMV retinitis in most cases, but there is generally not much resolution of existing damage.

Close ophthalmologic follow-up is needed to monitor for breakthrough progression of disease that may require repeat induction dosing, an increase in maintenance dose, or changing to foscarnet.

Most clinicians use ganciclovir for other severe CMV infections as warranted, often without continued maintenance dosing.

Foscarnet: Foscarnet is approved for the treatment of CMV retinitis. It is about as effective as ganciclovir and 1 study showed a life-prolonging effect compared to ganciclovir although the reasons for this are unclear.

The dose of foscarnet must be based on renal function. A 24-hour urine collection to measure creatinine clearance rather than relying solely on calculated values is recommended.

For those patients with good renal function (CrCl > 1.6 ml/min/kg) the following doses are used:

Induction: 60 mg/kg IV Q 8 hrs for 14–21 days
Maintenance: 90–120 mg/kg IV daily

The most common side effects are renal impairment, electrolyte abnormalities (especially calcium), fever, nausea, anemia, vomiting, headache, and seizures.

Renal function **and** electrolytes (calcium, magnesium, potassium, and phosphorus) must be closely monitored (see Chapter 15).

There has been at least 1 reported case of CMV resistance to foscarnet.

REFERENCES

Drew WL: Cytomegalovirus infection in patients with AIDS. *Clin Inf Dis* 1992;**14:**608.

Gallant JE, Moore RD, Richman DD: Incidence and natural history of cytomegalovirus disease in patients with advanced human immunodeficiency virus disease treated with zidovudine. *JID* 1992; **166:**1223.

Goodgame RW: Gastrointestinal cytomegalovirus disease. *Ann Int Med* 1993;**119:**924.

Jacobsen MA et al: A dose-ranging study of daily maintenance intravenous foscarnet therapy for cytomegalovirus retinitis in AIDS. *JID* 1993;**168:**444.

Kim YS, Hollander H: Polyradiculopathy due to cytomegalovirus: Report of two cases in which improvement occurred after prolonged therapy and review of the literature. *Clin Infect Dis* 1993;**17:**32.

Leport C et al: Cytomegalovirus resistant to foscarnet: Clinicovirologic correlation in a patient with human immunodeficiency virus. (Letter) *J Infect Dis* 1993;**168:**1329.

Studies of ocular complications of AIDS research group. Mortality in patients with the acquired immunodeficiency syndrome treated with either foscarnet or ganciclovir for cytomegalovirus retinitis. *N Engl J Med* 1992;**326:**213.

HERPES SIMPLEX

Herpes simplex (HSV) is a common sexually transmitted disease, which in HIV-infected patients may become chronic or persistent. In the immunocompetent person HSV is generally self-limited. As the immune system deteriorates, the frequency and severity of the lesions increases. Local lesions may become invasive and quite destructive and lose their characteristic appearance. Disseminated disease may be life-threatening. HSV is often divided into HSV-1 and HSV-2, however, this distinction has little clinical significance in HIV-infected people.

Presentation

Symptoms: The most common sites of involvement are genital, rectal, orolabial, and esophageal. The lesions generally begin as a painful vesicular eruption and progress to ulcerations. Pain is the primary complaint, but there also may be mild constitutional symptoms. The ulcers generally begin to heal within 7–14 days. In the immunocompromised, the lesions may persist much longer. Occasionally, the ulcerations become invasive; this is especially common in the rectal area. Aseptic meningitis or encephalitis may complicate localized disease.

Physical Findings: Orolabial–Vesicular eruptions may occur on the lips, tongue, and oral mucosa. Adenopathy may also be present.

Genital–Lesions may occur on any of the genitalia. The early vesicular lesions progress to multiple ulcers. Inguinal adenopathy and dysuria are often present.

Rectal–Rectal lesions may be minimal and similar to genital lesions, or they may be very severe, painful, and invasive. HSV is the most common cause of severe rectal lesions in HIV-infected patients. There is an increasing incidence of rectal malignancies in HIV-infected people and, therefore, a definitive diagnosis is desirable.

Diagnosis

A history of recurrent vesicular or ulcerative lesions is often obtained and if present, strongly suggests HSV. Tzanck smears will establish Herpes virus infection but do not distinguish between Herpes simplex and zoster. Viral culture is the definitive examination and is easily obtained by scraping the base of an ulcer or unroofing a vesicle, scraping the base with a swab and placing the swab in viral culture material. Immunofluorescence studies are also available.

Treatment

Oral acyclovir at a dose of 200 mg PO Q 4 hours 5 times daily for 10–14 days generally aids in resolution of the lesions. Severe lesions often require longer courses or higher doses. Disseminated disease may respond to higher PO doses (up to 800 mg 5 times daily) or IV acyclovir.

Patients with frequent recurrences may benefit from suppressive doses of acyclovir. Most patients do not have recurrences when taking 200 mg PO TID or 400 mg PO BID. Acyclovir is safe at this dose for long periods of time. One concern with prolonged use is the development of acyclovir-resistant HSV. This has been reported late in HIV disease and after prolonged use of acyclovir. Acyclovir resistant herpes usually responds to foscarnet 40 mg/kg IV TID. It is of interest that outbreaks of herpes that follow an acyclovir-resistant infection are often sensitive to acyclovir.

In addition to oral acyclovir, severe rectal disease is treated with topical silver sulfadiazine (do not use in patients with sulfa allergy) to prevent superinfection and protect the damaged skin. Topical acyclovir does not seem to be of significant value in the treatment of HSV.

REFERENCES

Englund JA et al: Herpes simplex virus resistant to acyclovir. *Ann Int Med* 1990;**112:**416.

Hardy DW: Foscarnet treatment of acyclovir-resistant herpes simplex virus infection in patients with acquired immunodeficiency syndrome: Results of a controlled, randomized, regimen comparative trial. *Am J Med* 1992;**92 2A:**S30.

Zuger A: Recurrent genital herpes in an HIV-infected woman. *AIDS Clinical Care* 1993;**5**:20.

HISTOPLASMOSIS

Histoplasma capsulatum (histo) is a fungus endemic to the South Central United States and South America. It is found in soil in spore form. When contaminated soil is disturbed, the spores may be inhaled where they germinate into the yeast form and spread via the blood throughout the body. Immunocompetent hosts generally contain the infection primarily in the lungs and develop immunity within 2 weeks. It appears that after infection, some viable organisms remain intracellularly, which in immunocompromised patients may result in "reactivation infection." Primary infection of immunocompromised individuals is also a possibility.

Presentation

Symptoms: The symptoms of histoplasmosis are reflective of the diffuse invasive nature of the infection. Fever, weight loss, skin lesions, adenopathy, respiratory complaints, cough, and hepatosplenomegaly are common. Meningitis and cerebritis are rarely seen.

Physical Findings: There are no specific physical findings. The CXR may be normal in a substantial number of patients with disseminated disease.

Diagnosis

Identification of the fungus in tissue specimens or in culture provides the definitive diagnosis. Bone marrow, blood, lymph nodes, lungs, and skin are all commonly infected tissues that should be examined and biopsied. Serologic tests for histoplasmosis are available. Complement fixation tests are reliable when positive, but may be negative in up to 30% of infected people. A new radioimmunoassay for the detection of a histo polysaccharide antigen, may be more sensitive. Skin testing has no role in diagnosis.

Treatment

Patients with disseminated histoplasmosis disease require intensive induction treatment with amphotericin. The total dose of amphotericin required is yet unknown, but some experts have used up to 2.5 grams. Maintenance or suppressive therapy is then required. Amphotericin is currently recommended for maintenance, but there have been good results with itraconazole (200 mg PO BID) in early studies. Consultation with knowledgeable specialists is recommended.

REFERENCES

Sarosi GA, Johnson PC: Disseminated histoplasmosis in patients infected with human immunodeficiency virus. *Clin Inf Dis* 1992;**14:**S60.

Wheat J et al: Prevention of relapse of histoplasmosis with itraconazole in patients with the acquired immunodeficiency syndrome. *Ann Int Med* 1993;**118:**610.

Wheat LJ et al: Histoplasmosis relapse in patients with AIDS: Detection using histoplasma capsulatum variety capsulatum antigen levels. *Ann Int Med* 1991;**115:**936.

KAPOSI'S SARCOMA

Kaposi's Sarcoma (KS) is a malignancy believed to originate in vascular or lymphatic endothelial cells. It is fairly common in HIV-infected patients. The cause of KS is unknown, however, epidemiologic evidence points toward an infectious agent.

Presentation

Symptoms: KS is generally first noted in the skin or oral cavity. At first presentation, the lesions are small and not painful. The course of KS is quite variable with some patients developing new lesions slowly and others fairly quickly developing disease throughout the body. The GI tract, lungs, lymphatics and genitals are common sites of involvement. GI disease is generally not symptomatic but may cause dysphagia, bleeding, diarrhea and malabsorption. Oral lesions may become painful or cause problems with eating. Pulmonary disease can be confused with PCP. Pulmonary disease is quite worrisome as it may rapidly interfere with respiratory function and is often fatal. Lymphatic involvement may result in debilitating lymphedema.

Physical Findings: Cutaneous or oral KS generally presents as painless nodules or macules, which are usually pigmented red, purple, or brown. Lymphatic disease may be severe with resultant lymphedema. Pulmonary disease generally presents with respiratory distress and pleural effusions are common.

Diagnosis

Punch biopsy of cutaneous lesions is the easiest method of diagnosis. Bronchoscopy is generally required for pulmonary diagnosis, however KS is suggested when a gallium scan is negative and a thallium pulmonary scan is positive.

Treatment

KS follows a variable course depending on the stage of HIV disease. Individuals may have only limited cutaneous disease while others have more extensive cutaneous disease and may progress to fatal pulmonary or other visceral disease. The psychologic damage of a disfiguring malignancy in addition to HIV-infection must be considered. Careful observation and patient reassurance is recommended for limited disease but moderate or bulky disease should be treated.

The treatment for KS is divided into 2 categories: (1) treatment of local lesions and (2) systemic therapy for progressive disseminated disease.

Local Lesions: Lesions that are small and few in number

are generally treated only if they are painful or causing cosmetic problems. Radiotherapy, cryotherapy, and intralesional injections with vinblastine are all useful for local lesions. Most lesions respond well to these therapies initially, but recurrence is common.

Progressive Cutaneous and Disseminated Disease: Chemotherapy has been the standard approach to disseminated disease. Several agents (vinblastine, vincristine, bleomycin, adriamycin and etoposide) are used in a variety of regimens. Liposomal encapsulated daunorubicin and adriomycin are under evaluation and may represent an important new approach to therapy. Systemic alfa-interferon, alone or in combination with zidovudine, is effective in patients with limited cutaneous disease and CD4 cell count > 100–200. Consultation with knowledgeable specialists is indicated.

REFERENCES

Beral V et al: Kaposi's sarcoma among persons with AIDS: A sexually transmitted infection? *Lancet* 1990;**335**:123.

Myskowski PL: Kaposi's sarcoma: Where do we go from here? *Arch Derm* 1993;**129**:1320.

Presant CA, Scolaro M, Kennedy P: Liposomal daunorubicin treatment of HIV-associated Kaposi's sarcoma. *Lancet* 1993;**341**:1242.

Tappero JW et al: Cryotherapy for cutaneous Kaposi's sarcoma associated with acquired immune deficiency syndrome: A phase 2 trial. *J Acq Imm Def* 1991:4839.

Zuger A: Cough in a patient with Kaposi's sarcoma. *AIDS Clinical Care* 1992;**4**:31.

HIV-RELATED LYMPHOMA

The relationship between immunocompromise and lymphoma has been observed for many years. In 1985, the CDC expanded the definition of AIDS to include HIV-infected people with high-grade B-cell non-Hodgkin's lymphoma. Patients with primary B-cell lymphoma of CNS also meet criteria for AIDS. Epstein-Barr virus has been found to be associated with AIDS related CNS lymphoma.

Presentation

Symptoms: Lymphoma in HIV-infected patients is commonly extranodal. The most common sites are: the GI tract, CNS, bone marrow, liver, lungs, and pleura. Unusual sites of involvement include: the heart, rectum, gingiva, Waldeyer's ring, and the bile duct. Symptoms are related to the organ system involved. Unfortunately, early symptoms may be nonspecific and thus nondirective. Lymphadenopathy is common in HIV and is of greatest concern when asymmetric or rapidly enlarging nodes are present. Lymphoma must be in the differential of hepatic or GI symptoms or abnormalities. CNS lymphoma presents with altered mental status, headaches, or focal neurologic findings.

Physical Findings: Findings are dependent on organ system involved. New asymmetric adenopathy or rapidly enlarging nodes should be of particular concern. Anorectal complaints and particularly the presumptive diagnosis of anorectal abscess should spark the consideration of lymphoma. Adenopathy of the abdominal or pulmonary nodes may be lymphoma, particularly in the absence of other diagnosis (eg, MAC may cause abdominal adenopathy).

Diagnosis

Biopsy is generally required for diagnosis. CNS lymphoma is first found on CT or MRI. The lesions may be single or multiple and hypodense, isodense, or ring enhancing with some degree of mass effect. The radiologic appearance is not diagnostic and the differential includes fungal or bacterial abscesses and toxoplasmosis. Brain biopsy is required for definitive diagnosis. Some clinicians will empirically treat patients with mass lesions for toxoplasmosis. If patients do not show clinical and radiographic improvement over a 1–2 week period, a definitive diagnosis via brain biopsy should be obtained. With this approach, brain biopsy is required only in patients with negative serology or who do not respond to empiric therapy.

CSF examination may yield neoplastic cells in a small percentage of patients. An Italian study suggests that PCR (polymease chain reaction) testing of CSF for Epstein-Barr virus DNA may be useful in diagnosing CNS lymphoma in AIDS patients.

Treatment

CNS disease is treated with whole-brain radiotherapy. Neurologic signs and symptoms may respond to systemic corticosteroids. The prognosis is poor.

Peripheral lymphomas may be treated with a variety of chemotherapeutic regimens (CHOP, BACOP, and MBACOD). The mean survival with chemotherapy is approximately 6 months. There is some evidence that aggressive chemotherapy may actually shorten survival time. The decision to treat HIV-related lymphoma is difficult. Patients with CD4 counts of > 100 and good performance status may live a longer life with chemotherapy while those with poor performance status and low CD4 counts may actually do worse with chemotherapy. Because of the questions surrounding optimal treatment, consultation with knowledgeable specialists is suggested.

REFERENCES

Cinque P et al: Epstein-Barr virus DNA in cerebrospinal fluid from patients with AIDS-related primary lymphoma of the central nervous system. *Lancet* 1993;**342:**398.

Levine AM: Epidemiology, clinical characteristics, and management of AIDS-related lymphoma. *Hematol Oncol Clin North Am* 1991;**5:**331.

MYCOBACTERIUM AVIUM COMPLEX

Mycobacterium avium Complex (MAC) infections occur late in the course of HIV infection, generally in those with < 50–100 CD4 cells. MAC is common and some autopsy series have found up to 50% of patients infected. Studies of death rates in patients with MAC indicate an increased mortality in those infected. Treatment of disseminated MAC can reduce the concentration and duration of bacteremia, and alleviate symptoms.

Presentation

Symptoms: Symptoms attributed to MAC infection are multiple and nonspecific. Fever, fatigue, chills, nightsweats, anorexia, weight loss, diarrhea, and abdominal pain are common in patients with MAC infection. These symptoms are obviously common to many HIV-related illnesses. In our experience, patients with < 50–100 CD4 cells, who have abdominal pain associated with diarrhea, and abdominal adenopathy are most likely to have MAC infection.

Physical Findings: Hepatosplenomegaly and palpable abdominal lymphadenopathy may be present. Anemia is present in cases of marrow involvement. Abdominal films and especially CT scans generally reveal marked lymphadenopathy.

Diagnosis

The diagnosis of MAC infection is based on the isolation of the organism (by culture) from the blood, bone marrow, or tissue (lymph node, liver). Special techniques are used to improve the yield and shorten the recovery time for mycobacterium growth. Blood cultures for MAC should be ordered when HIV-infected patients present with signs or symptoms compatible with mycobacterial infection.

Positive stool or sputum cultures may represent either MAC colonization or infection. The decision to treat these patients is generally based on the presence of symptoms consistent with MAC infection or a CD4 count of < 50.

Treatment

Combination therapy is required to treat MAC. There are published data regarding successful treatment regimens for

MAC. Amakicin, azithromycin, ciprofloxacin, clarithromycin, clofazamine, ethambutol, ofloxacin, rifabutin, and rifampin are all active against MAC to some degree. Clarithromycin has been approved in combination with other antimycobacterial drugs for the treatment of MAC.

The current practice is to use combination therapy including a macrolide such as clarithromycin and 1 or 2 other active agents to prevent drug resistance. Combinations that are potentially effective include clarithromycin with ethambutol and/or clofazamine. Other potentially useful agents include rifampin, ciprofloxacin, amikacin, and azithromycin. Medications and doses are listed below. If intolerance to a particular drug develops, consider substituting with another from the list.

> Amikacin 7.5 mg/kg/day IV/IM QD for up to 8 weeks (generally reserved for very ill patients or those failing oral regimens)
> Azithromycin 500–900 mg PO QD
> Ciprofloxacin 750 mg PO BID
> Clarithromycin 500 mg PO BID (1000 mg BID may be used if the patient does not respond to 500 mg BID)
> Clofazamine 100–200 mg PO QD
> Ethambutol 25 mg/kg/day for 6 weeks and then 15 mg/kg (max 1200 mg) PO QD
> Rifampin 300 mg PO QD

The PO medications are continued for life. These drugs have considerable toxicities that must be monitored. There are also many significant interactions between these drugs and other drugs commonly used in HIV-infection.

The goals of treatment include symptomatic improvement (usually within 4–6 weeks) and sterilization of the blood.

Prophylaxis

Rifabutin has recently been approved for prophylaxis against MAC. A full discussion is found in Chapter 6, "Prophylaxis Against Opportunistic Infections."

REFERENCES

Chiu J, Nussbaum J, Bozzette S et al: Treatment of disseminated *Mycobacterium avium* complex infection in AIDS with amikacin, ethambutol, rifampin, and ciproflaxacin. *Ann Int Med* 1990; **113:**358.

Ellner JJ, Goldberger MJ, Parenti DM: *Mycobacterium avium* infection and AIDS: A therapeutic dilemma in rapid evolution. *J Infect Dis* 1991;**163:**1326.

Horsburgh CR: *Mycobacterium avium* complex infection in the acquired immunodeficiency syndrome. *N Engl J Med* 1991; **324:**1332.

Hoy J et al: Quadruple-drug therapy for *Mycobacterium avium* bacteremia in AIDS patients. *J Inf Dis* 1990;**161:**801.

Jacobson MA, Yajko D, Northfelt D: Randomized, placebo controlled trial of rifampin, ethambutol, and ciproflaxacin for AIDS patients with disseminated *Mycobacterium avium* complex infection. *J Infect Dis* 1993;**168:**112.

Jorup-Ronstrom C, Julander I, Petrini B: Efficacy of triple drug regimen of amikacin, ethambutol, and rifabutin in AIDS patients with symptomatic *Mycobacterium avium* complex infection. *J Infect* 1993;**26:**67.

Kemper CA et al: California Collaborative Treatment Group. Treatment of *Mycobacterium avium* complex bacteremia in AIDS with a four-drug oral regimen: Rifampin, ethambutol, clofazamine, and ciproflaxacin. *Ann Int Med* 1992;**116:**466.

Kerlikowske KM et al: Antimycobacterial therapy for disseminated *Mycobacterium avium* complex infection in patients with acquired immunodeficiency syndrome. *Arch Intern Med* 1992;**152:**813.

Lalla F, Maserati R, Scarpellini P et al: Clarithromycin-ciprofloxacin-amikacin for therapy of *Mycobacterium avium-Mycobacterium intracellulare* bactermia in patients with AIDS. *Antimicrob Agents Chemother* 1992;**36:**1567.

Nightingale SD et al: Incidence of *Mycobacterium avium*-intracellulare complex bacteremia in human immunodeficiency virus-positive patients. *J Infect Dis* 1992;**165:**1082.

Public Health Service Task Force on Prophylaxis and Therapy for *Mycobacterium Avium* Complex. Special Report: Recommendations on prophylaxis and therapy for disseminated *Mycobacterium avium* complex disease in patients infected with the human immunodeficiency virus. *N Engl J Med* 1993;**329:**898.

MYCOBACTERIUM TUBERCULOSIS (MTB)

HIV-infected individuals are at an increased risk for developing tuberculosis and MTB may be the first clinical manifestation of immunodeficiency. It is important that people with MTB be tested for HIV infection as therapy is altered by the diagnosis; conversely, it is important that HIV-infected individuals receive yearly tuberculin skin testing.

A relatively recent development is the increase in drug resistant MTB. MTB cases resistant to 1 or more drugs have been reported from all regions of the USA. Since 1990, 9 outbreaks of multiple drug-resistant MTB (MDRTB) have been investigated in hospitals and prisons. Among those cases of MDRTB, most occurred in HIV-infected individuals. The case fatality rate has been high, from 72–89% (when there was resistance to both INH and rifampin) and the interval between diagnosis and death has been short—within a range of 4–16 weeks.

Because poor compliance with prescribed treatment is a major cause of treatment failures and drug-resistant MTB, directly observed therapy (health care personnel observe while the patient ingests the medication) is assuming a larger role in ensuring adherence to a prescribed treatment regimen.

For purposes of clarification, an individual is considered to have tuberculosis infection, but no disease if a PPD is positive but cultures and CXR are negative. Tuberculosis with active disease is diagnosed if cultures are positive or if PPD and CXR are positive.

Presentation

Symptoms: The symptoms of MTB are generally nonspecific and include fever, nightsweats, weight loss, cough, and hemoptysis. Extrapulmonary MTB occurs frequently in HIV-infected individuals (often with coexistent pulmonary MTB). Symptoms will vary according to site of infection.

Physical Findings: Lungs, pleura, lymph nodes, bone marrow, peripheral blood, GI and GU tracts, brain, bone, skin, soft tissues, and pericardium have been documented as sites of infection. Findings vary with the organ system involved.

Diagnosis

PPD and anergy testing with at least 2 antigens should be performed annually on HIV-infected individuals unless they have a history of a positive PPD, have had a BCG vaccination < 5 years ago, or have been anergic on 2 consecutive testings.

Five tuberculin units (TU) of purified protein derivative (PPD)-tuberculin should be administered using the Mantoux method (0.1 ml administered intradermally).

Anergy testing may be performed using mumps antigen, *Candida* antigen, or tetanus toxoid (other antigens have also been used). Mumps antigen is the only standardized and licensed antigen for anergy testing. *Candida* antigen at 1:100 or 1:500 dilutions has been used. Tetanus toxoid in 1:5 dilution (with phenol-buffered diluent) has been used. All of the above antigens should be administered by the Mantoux method.

PPD and 2 or more controls should be administered at the same time and read at 48–72 hours after administration. Any amount of induration to mumps, *Candida,* or tetanus is considered positive. Erythema alone is not considered evidence of delayed type hypersensitivity responsiveness.

An individual who responds to 1 or more of the controls (mumps, *Candida,* tetanus) and does not respond to the PPD is considered to be PPD-negative and has probably not been exposed or infected with MTB. An individual who does not respond to any of the skin tests is considered anergic and MTB exposure or infection cannot be excluded. Anergy may occur in 10% of HIV-infected individuals with CD4 counts > 500 and up to 80% or more in patients with CD4 counts < 50.

PPD: 5 mm of induration or more is considered positive in HIV-infected persons.

CXR: Pulmonary MTB may reveal hilar or mediastinal adenopathy with or without pulmonary infiltrates, infiltrates in any lung zone with or without cavitation, pleural effusions, and a diffuse interstitial alveolar or miliary pattern. Atypical presentations may be confused with PCP or pulmonary disease secondary to other pathogens. Normal CXRs are occasionally seen.

Acid fast bacilli (AFB) staining and culture: Definitive diagnosis generally rests on the culture of MTB from infected fluids or tissue. Any HIV-infected patient with evidence of pulmonary disease should have at least 3 sputums sent for acid fast smear and culture. If adequate sputums cannot be obtained spontaneously or by sputum induction (using nebulized 3–5% hypertonic saline), bronchoscopy/bronchoalveolar lavage may be indicated. Culture of blood, lymph node tissue, stool, CSF, urine, bone marrow, etc may be indicated based on symptoms.

Drug susceptibility testing should be performed routinely on initial MTB isolates and if drug resistance is subsequently suspected. Results of susceptibility testing are now available within 2–5 weeks (ie, Bactec system) of obtaining specimens, although some regions may take as long as 2–4 months.

The finding of acid fast bacilli from any source requires prompt anti-tuberculosis treatment while awaiting culture, identification of the organism, and susceptibility test results if MTB is present.

Treatment

Positive PPD or history of positive PPD: HIV-infected individuals with latent MTB have a 7–10% risk of developing active tuberculosis per year.

Preventive therapy with INH 300 mg PO QD for 12 months should be initiated. HIV-infected people on INH should take pyridoxine 50 mg PO QD because of the risk of drug-induced neuropathy. Some experts continue to prescribe INH indefinitely.

Preventive therapy should be initiated only after CXR and clinical evaluation have excluded pulmonary or extrapulmonary MTB. If an HIV-infected patient is symptomatic and MTB cannot be excluded, starting full dose anti-tuberculosis therapy is recommended after cultures are obtained. If MTB is later excluded, then continue with INH alone for 12 months or INH plus rifampin for 6 months.

Exposure to MTB: In 2 recent outbreaks, 40% of HIV-infected individuals who were exposed to infectious MTB developed active tuberculosis within a few weeks to months.

PPD and 2 controls should be placed. (See next section if the patient is anergic.) For patients with a negative PPD, but high risk contact (immediate family members, close social contacts, or shared indoor environment for long periods), repeat the PPD at 12 weeks and initiate preventive (or anti-tuberculosis) therapy until then.

Patients with a positive PPD need either preventative therapy with INH or if active MTB is diagnosed, treatment should be initiated as below.

For patients exposed to MDRTB, consultation with experts is recommended. Consideration should be given to the contact history, the infectiousness (presence of cough; smear positive sputum) of the source case, the duration of exposure, and the closeness or proximity of the MDRTB exposure. Twelve months of preventive therapy with 2 or more drugs to which the microorganisms are sensitive should be considered, although no data are available on prophylaxis against MDRTB.

Anergic patients: Active MTB should be excluded as above.

Preventive INH for 12 months or more should be considered for those patients who are known to have been exposed to tuberculosis patients, or groups who belong to high risk groups, such as IDUs, homeless, prisoners, migrant laborers, or people born in Asia, Africa, Haiti, or Latin America where the prevalence of TB is greater than 10%.

Active MTB: It is recommended that clinicians work closely with local public health departments because many have developed contact tracking procedures and programs for directly observed therapy (DOT). Medication is often available at low or no cost to the patient. MTB is a reportable condition and the "Report of Verified Cases of Tuberculosis" has been revised to enable monitoring of drug susceptibility patterns in the USA.

To prevent the development of resistant organisms, multidrug therapy is required and patient compliance is essential. Noncompliance may be a factor in the development of resistant strains of MTB. Directly observed therapy has been recommended by the US Public Health Service for initial therapy in people with MTB. It is believed that HIV-infected patients with tuberculosis should have directly observed therapy through completion of therapy.

Treat suspected and newly diagnosed MTB in adults and children with 1 of 3 possible options (medication doses must be higher for intermittent therapy; see Table 8–1):

A. INH (with pyridoxime) plus rifampin plus pyrazinamide plus either ethambutol OR streptomycin daily for 8 weeks, followed by INH plus rifampin daily (or 2–3 times weekly under directly observed therapy) in areas where the INH resistance rate is potentially > 4%.
B. INH (with pyridoxime) plus rifampin plus pyrazinamide plus either ethambutol OR streptomycin daily for 2 weeks, followed by the same drugs 2 times weekly (by directly observed therapy) for 6 weeks, followed by INH plus rifampin 2 times weekly (under directly observed therapy).
C. INH (with pyridoxime) plus rifampin plus pyrazinamide plus either ethambutol OR streptomycin 3 times weekly under directly observed therapy. This regimen is not recommended.

- A minimum of 9–12 months of therapy is recommended. Treatment should continue until 6 months after follow-up cultures are negative. All initial isolates of MTB should be routinely tested for drug susceptibility. Send monthly sputums for AFB smear and culture until culture converts to negative unless otherwise indicated. Follow-up drug susceptibility testing is indicated if noncompliance is suspected or if response to therapy is atypical.

  If directly observed therapy is not employed, the use of rifamate (INH-rifampin combination) to prevent monotherapy and the development of drug resistance is recommended (Table 8–1).
- Ethambutol or streptomycin and pyrazinamide may be discontinued once susceptibility to INH and rifampin has been demonstrated. If drug susceptibility results are not available, ethambutol or streptomycin should be

TABLE 8–1: DOSAGE RECOMMENDATIONS FOR THE INITIAL TREATMENT OF MTB AMONG CHILDREN (≤12 YEARS) AND ADULTS

Drugs	Daily		2 times/week		3 times/week	
	Children	Adults	Children	Adults	Children	Adults
INH	10–20 mg/kg max 300 mg	5 mg/kg max 300 mg	20–40 mg/kg max 900 mg	15 mg/kg max 900 mg	20–40 mg/kg max 900 mg	15 mg/kg max 900 mg
Rifampin	10–20 mg/kg max 600 mg	10 kg/kg max 600 mg	10–20 mg/kg max 600 mg	10 mg/kg max 600 mg	10–20 mg/kg max 600 mg	10 mg/kg max 600 mg
Pyrazinamide	15–30 mg/kg max 2 gm	15–30 mg/kg max 2 gm	50–70 mg/kg max 4 gm	50–70 mg/kg max 4 gm	50–70 mg/kg max 3 gm	50–70 mg/kg max 3 gm
Ethambutol	15–25 mg/kg max 2.5 gm	5–25 mg/kg max 2.5 gm	50 mg/kg max 2.5 gm	50 mg/kg max 2.5 gm	25–30 mg/kg max 2.5 gm	25–30 mg/kg max 2.5 gm
Streptomycin	20–30 mg/kg max 1 gm	15 mg/kg max 1 gm	25–30 mg/kg max 1.5 gm	25–30 mg/kg max 1.5 gm	25–30 mg/kg max 1 gm	25–30 mg/kg max 1 gm

Adapted from Centers for Disease COntrol and Prevention. Initial Therapy for tuberculosis in the era of multidrug resistance. Recommendations of the Advisory Council for the Elimination of Tuberculosis. *MMWR* 1993;**42 (No. RR–7)**:1.

continued for the full course of treatment because of rapid disease progression if inadequate therapy is given (Table 8–1).
- Suspect MDRTB and consult with experts if the patient is symptomatic or smear or culture positive after 3 months. Patients who are failing treatment should be treated with additional medications after repeat cultures and susceptibility testing is done. **At least 2 drugs that the patient has never received before should be added** (based on drug susceptibility results when available). This may not be adequate if MDRTB is present.

  Proven MDRTB may require 6 or 7 medications. In areas where strains of MTB are commonly resistant to 2 or more agents, it may be necessary to begin HIV-infected patients on a 6-drug regimen based on local patterns of drug resistance. Specific MTB isolate drug susceptibilities should guide therapy in all proven MDRTB cases. Serum peak and trough levels may be used to optimize therapy.
- All of the medications used in the treatment of MTB have associated toxicities and interactions with other medications (ie, ketoconozole inhibits rifampin absorption). Frequent review of these toxicities and careful consideration of drug interactions is recommended.
- Liver function tests should be obtained baseline for patients on MTB medications and then at 3, 6, and 9 months (if abnormal, follow monthly LFTs). Patients should be instructed on symptoms of hepatitis (fever, abdominal pain, jaundice, and vomiting) and should be told to notify their physician promptly.
- CXR is recommended every 3 months unless there is a clinical change.

Prevention/Infection Control

Exercise a high level of suspicion and obtain CXRs and sputums for AFB smear and culture for all patients with pulmonary symptoms. HIV-infected patients with symptoms suggestive of MTB (such as respiratory symptoms or unexplained fever) or positive AFB in their sputum must be placed in AFB isolation until MTB is excluded (Table 8–2). Patients with sus-

TABLE 8–2. COMPARISON OF RESPIRATORY ISOLATION WITH AFB ISOLATION

	Respiratory Precautions	Acid Fast Bacilli Precautions
Criteria	Any patient with an infection that can be transferred by droplets through air.	All patients with positive AFB smear or culture. All patients with suspected tuberculosis.
Room	Private room with closed door	Private room with closed door. Negative air pressure ventilation. Ultraviolet lighting if possible.
Persons entering room	Wearing a mask is required before entering and must be removed after leaving patient room.	Particulate respirator put on before entering room and removed after leaving patient room.
Patient leaving room	Patient to wear mask upon being transported out of room. Not necessary for personnel transporting patient to wear mask.	Patient not to leave room unless necessary. If necessary, patient is to wear a properly fitted cone mask or valveless particulate respirator. A mask is not necessary for personnel transporting patient.
When to stop precautions		Patient may come off AFB isolation when there are at least 2 negative sputum smears obtained on different days.
Special instructions		Primary physicians may clear patients from AFB isolation if patient meets following criteria: A satisfactory clinical response has been reached, ie, patient no longer coughing, **or** reduction in number of AFB on repeat sputum smears, **or** culture identifies AFB as *Mycobacterium* other than tuberculosis.

Adapted from: Jackson Memorial Hospital Infection Control Manual

pected pulmonary MTB but 3 negative sputum smears, and patients with positive smears and presumably susceptible organisms should remain in AFB isolation for 2–3 weeks until there is a definite clinical and bacteriologic response. For patients with suspected resistant organisms, AFB isolation should be continued indefinitely or until at least 3 consecutive cultures are negative.

In clinics, coughing patients should wear masks, although their value is unproven. Ultraviolet germicidal irradiation and proper ventilation (when available) lessen the likelihood of tuberculosis transmission. Patients with suspected or proven MTB should be seen in separate areas.

Health care workers exposed to patients with cough should wear properly fitted masks. OSHA guidelines state that HEPA (high efficiency particulate air) filtration masks must be worn. However, no formal studies documenting their effectiveness have been done.

Consider frequent PPD testing for at-risk health care workers. Some experts recommend PPD testing every 6 months.

Prior to ordering pentamidine PCP prophylaxis, patients should be evaluated with PPD (and controls), CXR, and sputums (if indicated by symptoms).

REFERENCES

Braun M, Cote T, Rabkin C: Trends in death with tuberculosis during the AIDS era. *JAMA* 1993;**269**:2865.

Centers for Disease Control. National action plan to combat multidrug-resistant tuberculosis; Meeting the challenge of multidrug-resistant tuberculosis: Summary of a conference; Management of persons exposed to multidrug-resistant tuberculosis. *MMWR* 1992;**41 (No. RR–11)**:1.

Centers for Disease Control. Purified protein derivative (PPD)-tuberculin anergy and HIV Infection: Guidelines for anergy testing and management of anergic persons at risk of tuberculosis. *MMWR* 1991;**40 (No. RR–5)**:1.

Centers for Disease Control and Prevention. Initial therapy for tuberculosis in the era of multidrug resistance. Recommendations of the Advisory Council for the Elimination of Tuberculosis. *MMWR* 1993;**42 (No. RR–7)**:1.

Fischl M et al: Clinical presentation and outcome of patients with HIV infection and tuberculosis caused by multiple drug-resistant bacilli. *Ann Intern Med* 1992;**117:**184.

Iseman M: Treatment of multidrug-resistant tuberculosis. *NEJM* 1993;**329:**784.

Kornbluth R, McCutchan JA: Skin test responses as predictors of tuberculosis infection and of progression in HIV-infected persons. *Ann Intern Med* 1993;**119:**241.

Mahmoudi A, Iseman M: Pitfalls in the care of patients with tuberculosis: Common errors and their association with the acquisition of drug resistance. *JAMA* 1993;**270:**65.

Moreno S et al: Risk of developing tuberculosis among anergic patients infected with HIV. *Ann Intern Med* 1993;**119:**194.

OSHA Enforcement Policy Directive. October 8, 1993. CDC Guidelines for Environmental Control . . . Federal Register II, October 12, 1993.

PNEUMOCYSTIS CARINII

Pneumocystis carinii is a protozoan (or possibly a fungus) that infects the lungs causing fever, inflammation, and impaired gas exchange in immunocompromised people. *Pneumocystis carinii* pneumonia (PCP) is the most common opportunistic infection in untreated HIV-infected patients in the USA. Pneumocystis should be considered in all pneumonias in HIV-infected people.

Presentation

Symptoms: The onset of pneumocystis pneumonia is insidious with early, nonspecific symptoms of fever, fatigue, weight loss, diarrhea, and malaise. Cough, either nonproductive or productive of scant, thin, clear mucous is variable at the onset, but becomes more prominent later in disease. Shortness of breath and dyspnea on exertion are suggestive of PCP. In patients receiving pentamidine prophylaxis, the presentation is often subtle. Other organs may be involved and disseminated pneumocystis has been seen.

Physical findings: Tachypnea, fever, cyanosis (in severe PCP), wheezes, crackles, or rales may be present in PCP.

Diagnosis

CD4 cells: Generally CD4 counts are < 200 in patients with PCP. While not excluding PCP, counts > 200 suggest other pathogens.

CXR: Bilateral interstitial infiltrates are the classic radiologic finding. However, especially in early PCP, the CXR may be normal. Pleural effusions or adenopathy suggests other processes.

Arterial blood gases: These are important to obtain in individuals with suspected PCP because the ABG is often markedly abnormal despite a seemingly comfortable patient. An increased alveolar-artierial gradient (> 35 mm Hg) and pO_2 < 80 are suggestive of PCP.

LDH: Usually elevated, but this is a nonspecific finding.

Sputum induction: Induce sputum with 3% saline via ultrasonic nebulizer. Send for special stains and immunofluorescent studies. The percentage of positive results varies with the cytologist's training and experience. It is also advisable to send collected sputum for routine bacterial, AFB, and fungal studies.

Gallium scan: A diffuse pattern of pulmonary uptake is suggestive, but not diagnostic, of PCP. Gallium scanning is sometimes used when bronchoscopy is unavailable to make a presumptive diagnosis of PCP.

Bronchoscopy: Bronchoscopy with bronchoalveolar lavage or biopsy is extremely useful. A low threshold for bronchoscopy is indicated in HIV-infected patients given the wide range of pulmonary pathogens seen in the face of this infection.

Treatment

Mild disease: Outpatient oral therapy (as listed below) may be used if close follow-up is assured.

TMP/SMX: 15–20 mg/kg TMP component PO daily divided QID

- or -

Dapsone 100 mg PO QD and TMP 20 mg/kg PO daily divided QID (Check G6PD level when indicated)

- or -

Atovaquone 750 mg TID (take with food)

- or -

Clindamycin 450 mg PO QID and primaquine 30 mg PO QD

Clinical trials have found atovaquone to be associated with more treatment failures and a lower survival rate than TMP/SMX. There is, however, less toxicity with atovaquone compared to TMP/SMX.

Treatment should continue for 14–21 days. TMP/SMX levels may be measured and may be used to guide dosing.

Immediate admission to the hospital is recommended if any deterioration occurs.

Moderate to severe disease: Hospitalization is recommended for supplemental oxygen, close monitoring, and IV TMP/SMX, pentamidine, or trimetrexate (which has recently been approved by the FDA). Several new therapies are under investigation for PCP treatment in patients intolerant of TMP/SMX. These include clindamycin with primaquine as well as atovaquone and eflornithine.

Treatment with corticosteroids have been shown to decrease mortality in moderate to severe PCP. The indications for corticosteroids are a pO_2 of < 70 or an alveolar-arterial gradient of > 35 mm Hg. Prednisone is given at 40 mg PO BID day 1–5, 40 mg PO QD day 6–10, and 20 mg PO day 11–21.

REFERENCES

Hughes W et al: Comparison of atovaquone (566C80) with trimethoprim-sulfamethoxazole to treat *Pneumocystis carinii* pneumonia in patients with AIDS. *N Engl J Med* 1993;**328:**1521.

Masuer H: Prevention and treatment of pneumocystis pneumonia. *N Engl J Med* 1992;**327:**1853.

Medina I et al: Oral therapy for *Pneumocystis carinii* pneumonia in the acquired immunodeficiency syndrome. *N Engl J Med* 1990;**323:**776.

National Institutes of Health–University of California expert panel for corticosteroids as adjunctive therapy for pneumocystis pneumonia.

Consensus statement on the use of corticosteroids as adjunctive therapy for pneumocystis pneumonia in the acquired immunodeficiency syndrome. *N Engl J Med* 1990;**323:**1500.

Toma E et al: Clindamycin/primaquine versus trimethoprim-sulfamethoxazole as primary therapy for *Pneumocystis carinii* pneumonia in AIDS: A randomized, double-blind pilot trial. *Clin Inf Dis* 1993;**17:**178.

Weinberger SE: Recent advances in pulmonary medicine. *N Engl J Med* 1993;**328:**1462.

PROGRESSIVE MULTIFOCAL LEUKOENCEPHALOPATHY

Progressive multifocal leukoencephalopathy (PML) is an opportunistic infection caused by the JC virus. (Probably most often resulting from the reactivation of a latent viral infection.) This human papovavirus causes selective demyelination of the white matter of the brain. PML develops in approximately 4–5% of HIV-infected individuals. It should be considered in cases of progressive neurologic disease in HIV-infected patients.

Presentation

Symptoms: The onset is generally subacute with slowly progressive neurologic dysfunction. Dementia, visual deficits, hemiparesis, ataxia, difficulties with speech and language, abnormal gait, sensory deficits, or other focal deficits may occur. Altered consciousness resulting from brain swelling does not occur.

Physical Findings: Focal neurologic deficits are apparent. Patients are generally afebrile. Dementia may occur.

Diagnosis

CT or MRI: These studies reveal focal or diffuse lesions in the white matter typically without mass effect or contrast enhancement. MRI is more sensitive than CT. The white matter lesions observed with PML may be mimicked by those seen with

HIV encephalopathy.

Brain Biopsy: The definitive diagnosis rests on brain biopsy.

CSF: The CSF is usually normal, and it may be helpful in excluding other infections or conditions.

Treatment

There is no proven therapy for this disease. IV and intrathecal cytosine arabinoside (cytarabine) have been reported effective in some AIDS patients often weeks to months after initiation of treatment. Although rare cases of spontaneous sustained remission have been reported, especially in those with CD4 counts > 200 or those taking high dose zidovudine, the prognosis is poor with the mean length of survival < 6 months after onset of neurologic symptoms.

REFERENCES

Berger JR et al: Progressive multifocal leukoencephalopathy associated with human immunodeficiency virus infection. *Ann Intern Med* 1987;**107:**78.

Berger JR, Major EO: Progressive multifocal leukoencephalopathy. In: *Textbook of AIDS Medicine.* Broder S, Merigan T, Bolognesi D (editors). Williams & Wilkins, 1994.

Lidman C et al: Progressive multifocal leukoencephalopathy in AIDS. (Letter). *AIDS* 1991;**5:**1039.

Nicoli F et al: Efficacy of cytarabine in progressive multifocal leukoencephalopathy in AIDS. (Letter). *Lancet* 1992;**339:**306.

Portegies P et al: Response to cytarabine in progressive multifocal leukoencephalopathy in AIDS. (Letter). *Lancet* 1991;**337:**680.

SYPHILIS

The treatment of syphilis in HIV-infected patients is controversial. Although there is some evidence to the contrary, there has been documentation of an increased incidence of treatment failures and a more rapid progression to neurosyphilis in HIV-infected individuals with syphilis. Patients with syphilis should be tested for HIV infection and HIV-infected individuals should receive testing for syphilis. Consider neurosyphilis in HIV-infected patients with neurologic disease.

Presentation

Symptoms: Chancre, fever, or rash may occur. Altered mental status, facial palsy, hemiplegia or hemiparesis, ocular symptoms, and hearing loss may occur in neurosyphilis.

Physical Findings: Typical and atypical presentations include hepatitis, iritis, retinitis, lymphadenopathy, aortitis, meningitis, or encephalitis.

Diagnosis

RPR and FTA: These serologic tests are accurate for the majority of HIV-infected individuals coinfected with syphilis. Rarely, serology has been found to be negative in patients with confirmed secondary syphilis. Thus, when syphilis is suspected but serology is negative, consider darkfield microscopy or direct fluorescent antibody staining of exudate.

Lumbar Puncture: Neurosyphilis is confirmed with a positive CSF serology (VDRL) in the absence of gross blood contamination.

Neurosyphilis is considered **probable** given a reactive serum FTA; a negative CSF VDRL, but cell count > 20 or protein > 60 with no other explanations for CSF findings; and neurologic or ophthalmologic abnormalities consistent with syphilis. Neurosyphilis is considered **possible** given a reactive serum FTA; a negative CSF VDRL, but cell count > 20 or protein > 60 with no other explanations for CSF findings; and no neurologic manifestations. Neurosyphilis is unusual in the absence of a reactive serum VDRL or RPR.

Treatment

Primary and Secondary Syphilis of less than 1 year Duration: Benzathine Penicillin G 2.4 million units IM once a week for 3 weeks is recommended.

Follow the patient with clinical examinations and serology monthly for 3 months and then every 3 months. Titers for RPR or VDRL should decrease 4-fold (that is, 2 dilutions, ie, 1:16 to 1:4) within 3 months and are usually nonreactive by 12 months.

If titers fail to decrease or if titers increase, treat as syphilis of > 1 year duration.

The CDC recommends penicillin regimens for all stages of syphilis in HIV-infected individuals. They recommend skin testing for penicillin allergy followed by desensitization, if necessary.

Other experts have recommended Doxycycline 100 mg po BID for 28 days as alternative treatment.

Syphilis of greater than 1 year Duration or Latent Syphilis or Neurosyphilis: A CSF examination is recommended for HIV-infected patients with syphilis present for over 1 year or latent syphilis. If lumbar puncture is not clinically feasible, these patients should be treated for presumed neurosyphilis with

> Aqueous PCN G 2–4 million units IV Q 4 hours for 10 days
>
> -or -
>
> Procaine PCN G 2.4 million units IM QD with probenecid 500 mg PO QID for 10 days.

Ceftriaxone 1–2 grams/day for 10–14 days has been studied. It does not appear to offer any advantage over penicillin unless the patient is allergic to penicillin.

Patients with documented neurosyphilis should have repeat CSF examination at 6 and 12 months. Because of HIV alone, the cell count may never normalize however a decline below 20 cells/μg should be expected.

REFERENCES

Berger JR, Levy RM: The neurologic complications of human immunodeficiency virus infection. *Med Clin North Am* 1993;**77**:1.

Centers for Disease Control and Prevention. 1993 Sexually transmitted diseases treatment guidelines. *MMWR* 1993;**42 (No. RR–14)**:37.

Dowell ME et al: Response of latent syphilis or neurosyphilis to ceftriaxone therapy in persons infected with human immunodeficiency virus. *Am J Med* 1992;**93**:481.

Drugs for AIDS and associated infections. *The Medical Letter* 1993;**35**:79.

Gourevitch MN et al: Effects of HIV infection on the serologic manifestations and response to treatment of syphilis in intravenous drug users. *Ann Int Med* 1993;**118**:350.

Hicks CB et al: Seronegative secondary syphilis in a patient with the human immunodeficiency virus (HIV) with Kaposi's sarcoma: A diagnostic dilemma. *Ann Intern Med* 1987;**107**:492.

Musher DM, Hamill RJ, Baugn RE: Effect of human immunodeficiency virus (HIV) infection on the course of syphilis and on the response to treatment. *Ann Int Med* 1990;**113**:872.

THROMBOCYTOPENIA

Thrombocytopenia may occur with HIV infection. Recent data have been presented that suggest that in HIV there is diminished platelet production and decreased platelet survival possibly resulting from the direct infection of megakaryocytes.

Presentation

Symptoms: The presentation is generally made on laboratory testing. Bruising easily, epistaxis, gingival, or rectal bleeding may be present. Platelet counts as low as 10,000 are often without symptoms.

Physical Findings: Petechiae and ecchymoses may be seen.

Diagnosis

Platelet counts of < 100,000 define thrombocytopenia. Bone marrow biopsy often reveals decreased megakaryocytes.

Treatment

There are several possible approaches to the management of thrombocytopenia in HIV:

1. Zidovudine
2. Prednisone
3. Intravenous gamma globulin
4. Splenectomy
5. Danazol
6. Low dose splenic irradiation
7. No therapy

The above listed approaches have met with some success. A conservative approach with careful observation and education for nonbleeding patients is recommended. Zidovudine, if tolerated, should be initiated because it has been found to increase platelet production in HIV-infected patients with and without thrombocytopenia. Patients with dangerously low platelet counts (< 10,000) or significant bleeding should be hospitalized. In hospitalized patients, IV gamma-globulin followed by platelet transfusion generally results in rapid correction. Prednisone is then begun, and the patient is discharged. Outpatient follow-up must be close, and the goal should be to taper the prednisone to the lowest possible dose that will keep the patient symptom-free and the platelet count > 15,000.

REFERENCES

Ballem PJ: Kinetic studies of the mechanism of thrombocytopenia in patients with human immunodeficiency virus infection. *N Engl J Med* 1992;**327:**1779.

Needleman SW, Sorace J, Poussin-Rosillo H: Low-dose splenic irradiation in the treatment of autoimmune thrombocytopenia in HIV-infected patients. *Ann Int Med* 1992;**116:**310.

Rarick MU et al: The long-term use of zidovudine in patients with severe immune-mediated thrombocytopenia secondary to infection with HIV. *AIDS* 1991;**5:**1357.

TOXOPLASMA GONDII

Toxoplasma gondii is a protozoan, which causes only a mild or even asymptomatic infection when it infects normal hosts. Cats and other animals serve as a reservoir for the organism that is spread to humans via ingestion of contaminated soil, water, or food, especially raw or undercooked meat. In the USA, it is believed that approximately 50% of the population has been infected with *Toxoplasma.* Toxoplasmosis can cause disease in immunosuppressed people by reactivation of latent infection or by new infection.

HIV-infected individuals have sometimes been advised to avoid cats and other pets owing to the risk of transmission of zoonotic infections. While proper hygiene is recommended, current data suggest that pet ownership need not be discouraged.

Presentation

Symptoms: Intracranial disease is the most common site of infection. Headaches, confusion, fevers, lethargy, seizures, and poor coordination or gait are the most common presenting symptoms. The onset of symptoms may be slow and insidious or rapid and dramatic.

Physical Findings: Focal neurologic changes (hemiparesis, ataxia, cranial nerve palsies, sensory deficits, aphasia, and hemianopia) are the most common signs. Aside from neurologic abnormalities, toxoplasmosis can also affect the eye, causing chorioretinitis. Other organ systems may also be affected (ie, lungs, heart, and liver).

Diagnosis

MRI or CT Scan: MRI is believed to be more sensitive than CT. When CT is performed, lesions are most evident after double dose delayed contrast study. Multiple ring-enhancing lesions may be noted, especially in the white matter or basal ganglia.

CSF Studies: LP should not be done prior to neuroimaging (to rule out mass effect and prevent herniation). Results may be normal or reveal increased protein and mild mononuclear pleocytosis. CSF toxoplasmosis IgG antibodies may be measured but negative studies do not exclude toxoplasmosis.

Serology: In symptomatic patients, serology may be useful in suggesting toxoplasmosis, however a negative serology cannot be used to reliably exclude toxoplasmic encephalitis.

Brain biopsy: Generally, therapy for toxoplasmosis is given prior to brain biopsy. Early biopsy should be considered if toxoplasmosis serology is nonreactive or only a single lesion is present on neuroimaging.

Treatment

Treatment does not kill tissue cysts from latent infection; therefore, life-long suppressive therapy is required.

Initial Treatment: Sulfadiazine 75 mg/kg PO loading dose followed by 100 mg/kg/day (6–8 grams) divided in 2–4 doses. (Clindamycin 600 mg IV or PO every 6 hours in cases of sulfa allergy)

- and -

Pyrimethamine 100 mg PO QD for 2 days as a loading dose followed by 50–100 mg/day in one dose

- also -

Folinic acid 10–20 mg PO daily is recommended.

Symptomatic relief should occur within 2 weeks and improvement is evident by 1 month. Treatment should continue for 6–9 weeks or until clinical and radiologic resolution followed by suppressive treatment.

Some recent small studies suggest that for patients unable to tolerate or unresponsive to standard therapy, combination dapsone (100 mg/day) and pyrimethamine (50 mg/day) or azithromycin (1800 mg PO followed by 1200 mg/day for 6 weeks followed by 600 mg/day) and pyrimethamine (50 mg/day) or atovaquone (750 mg QID with food) may be an alternative to the above regimens.

Suppressive Treatment: Pyrimethamine 50 mg PO 3 times weekly
- and -
Sulfadiazine 2–4 grams PO per day (divided QID) 3 times weekly (Clindamycin 300-450 mg PO Q 6-8 hours in cases of sulfa allergy)
- also -
Folinic acid 5–10 mg daily is recommended.

Recent research supports the recommendation that patients on suppressive treatment for toxoplasmosis need not receive additional medications for PCP prophylaxis.

At the time of this writing, sulfadiazine is no longer being manufactured in the USA. It is hoped that this situation will be remedied in the near future. To obtain sulfadiazine for treatment or maintenance therapy call the CDC at (404) 488-4928.

REFERENCES

Conti L: Companion animals for persons with HIV infection. *J Florida Med Assoc* 1993;**80:**817.

Dannemann B, McCutchan A, Israelski D: Treatment of toxoplasmic encephalitis in patients with AIDS: A randomized trial comparing pyrimethamine plus clindamycin to pyrimethamine plus sulfadiazine. *Ann Int Med* 1992;**116:**33.

Eighth International Conference on AIDS. Abstract No.POB 3277. Amsterdam, 1992.

Heald A, Flepp M, Chave JP: Treatment for cerebral toxoplasmosis protects against *Pneumocystis carinii* pneumonia in patients with AIDS. *Ann Int Med* 1991;**115:**760.

Kovavs JA: Efficacy of atovaquone in treatment of toxoplasmosis in patients with AIDS. *Lancet* 1992;**340:**637.

Luft BJ, Remington JS: Toxoplasmic encephalitis in AIDS. *Clin Inf Dis* 1992;**15:**211.

Luft BJ, Hafner R, Korzun AH: Toxoplasmic encephalitis in patients with the acquired immunodeficiency syndrome. *N Engl J Med* 1993;**329:**995.

Porter SB, Sande MA: Toxoplasmosis of the central nervous system in the acquired immunodeficiency syndrome. *N Engl J Med* 1992;**327:**1643.

Wallace MR et al: Cats and toxoplasmosis risk in HIV-infected adults. *JAMA* 1993;**269:**76.

VARICELLA ZOSTER

Varicella zoster (zoster) is caused by reactivation of the varicella zoster virus (VZV) latent in dorsal root ganglia. Zoster is common in HIV-infected people and may be the first clinical manifestation of immune compromise. The frequency of zoster in HIV infection is not known exactly; however, it is significant as indicated by a study in which 70% of 40 consecutive patients presenting with zoster were HIV-infected.

Presentation

Symptoms: Zoster begins with a prodromal phase of itching or deep aching pain. An erythematous rash then develops evolving rapidly to grouped vesicles. The emergence of the rash may be accompanied by constitutional symptoms of malaise, fatigue, headache, and fever.

Physical Findings: The classic physical finding is a vesicular rash confined to 1 dermatome. It is not uncommon for more than 1 adjacent dermatome to be involved. Rash involving nonadjacent dermatomes is diagnostic of disseminated zoster. There are several serious complications of zoster, ie, meningoencephalitis, cerebrovasculopathy, cranial nerve syndromes (Varicella zoster Ophthalmicus, Ramsey-Hunt Syndrome), and visceral involvement (pneumonitis, hepatitis etc).

Diagnosis

Generally, zoster is diagnosed on history and clinical findings. Tzanck smears will establish Herpes virus infection but do not distinguish between Herpes simplex and VZV. Viral cultures or direct immunofluorescence tests are definitive though rarely needed.

Treatment

The treatment of zoster has 3 primary goals: (1) control of pain, (2) minimize symptom duration, and (3) prevent complications such as postherpetic neuralgia (PHN) and disseminated zoster.

Pain control: The pain of zoster is generally controllable with mild to moderate analgesics.

Minimize symptom duration: Recent research has demonstrated that acyclovir given orally at a dose of 800 mg Q 4 hours 5 times daily or IV at 30 mg/kg/day will significantly decrease the severity and duration of symptoms. The best results are achieved when acyclovir is started as early as possible. The lesions of zoster may be quite extensive. Local care is needed to relieve itching and prevent secondary infection. Wet dressings or compresses of either aluminum acetate solution (Burow's solution) or tap water are soothing and may be applied 4–6 times daily. Lotions such as calamine may be used after the compresses. Ulcerated lesions may be treated with topical antibiotic creams or ointments. Silver sulfadiazine has good antibiotic and antifungal activity and also has been reported to be viracidal and thus may be a good choice.

Prevent complications: High dose oral acyclovir will generally prevent and treat the complications of zoster.

Disseminated or multidermatomal zoster in immunocompromised people may require hospitalization for intravenous acyclovir. Close follow-up of patients with HIV infection and zoster is recommended during the acute course, with careful observation for complications.

For patients with postherpetic neuralgia, topical capsaicin cream or low dose tricyclic antidepressants may be helpful.

Varicella resistant to acyclovir has been seen in patients who have been on long-term oral acyclovir. Ganciclovir or foscarnet may be indicated in resistant disease.

REFERENCES

Buchbinder SP et al: Herpes zoster and human immunodeficiency virus infection. *J Infect Dis* 1992;**166:**1153.

Friedman-Kien AE et al: Herpes zoster: A possible early clinical sign for the development of acquired immunodeficiency syndrome in high risk individuals. *J Am Acad Dermatol* 1986;**14:**1023.

9

Differential Diagnosis of Common Complaints in HIV-Infected Individuals

Dermatology

Dermatologic complaints are common in HIV-infected persons. Skin scrapings, cultures, and shave or punch biopsies may be necessary for diagnosis (Table 9–1, page 95).

Diarrhea

The approach to the HIV-infected individual with diarrhea begins with a thorough history to assess quality (including presence of blood or mucus), quantity, frequency of stool, relation to diet (eg, lactose or fat intake), and presence of fever or abdominal pain. A thorough physical examination with orthostatic vital signs and rectal exam with stool guaiac should also be performed (see chart on page 99).

Fatigue

As in other chronic debilitating illnesses, fatigue is a common complaint for HIV-infected individuals. One approach to the problem is outlined below. We recommend empathetic acknowledgment of the complaint and a discussion of the limitations of medical treatment (see chart on page 100).

Fever

The approach to the HIV-infected individual with fever begins with a thorough history and physical examination. If symptoms are present, workup should be directed accordingly. Consider that HIV-infected persons may have more than one process at the same time (see chart on page 101).

Hepatomegaly/Elevated Liver Enzymes

HIV-infected people frequently have elevated liver enzymes and possible causes may be multiple, as seen in the chart on page 102. The approach outlined in the chart focuses on HIV-specific causes, however, as in nonHIV-infected individuals hemochromatosis, Gilbert's disease, mononeucleosis, Wilson's disease, etc, may occur.

Headaches, Seizures, and Focal Neurologic Findings

A high degree of suspicion should greet any new neurologic finding in HIV-infected persons and a prompt and complete workup is generally indicated (see chart on page 103).

Odynophagia/Dysphagia

The most common cause for odynophagia/dysphagia in HIV infection is candida esophagitis (see chart on page 104).

Peripheral Neuropathy

Peripheral neuropathy is common in HIV-infected persons, especially those with CD4 counts < 100. Patients may describe burning, numbness, or aching feet (see chart on page 105).

Respiratory Complaints

Respiratory complaints include cough, shortness of breath or dyspnea on exertion, pleuritic chest pain, or hemotysis (see chart on page 106).

TABLE 9–1. DIAGNOSTIC APPROACHES TO DERMATOLOGIC MANIFESTATIONS IN HIV INFECTION

Description of Lesion	Possible Causes	Treatment
Folliculitis–inflammation of hair follicles with resultant papules/pustules	Staph or strep species (culture is diagnostic) HIV-associated eosinophilic folliculitis (pruritic papular eruption (PPE); "itchy red bump disease")–chronic (with exacerbations and remissions); face, head, trunk, and extremities may be involved.	Topical or systemic antibiotic Antihistamines and topical steroids may alleviate symptoms. Ultraviolet B light may be successful.
Papulosquamous dermatitis–characterized by scaly patches on skin	Seborrheic dermatitis–appears as "dandruff" in eyebrows, mustache, and nasolabial folds.	Selenium sulfide shampoo-wash affected areas Mild topical steroids with topical antifugal cream also useful.

(continued)

TABLE 9–1 *(continued)*

Description of Lesion	Possible Causes	Treatment
	Fungal and dermatophytes including candida, tineas, cryptococcus histoplasmosis, sporotrichosis.	Topical antifungals. Systemic antifungal treatment may be necessary.
	Xerotic eczema– widespread, dry, scaly, and pruritic.	Emollients.
	Psoriasis may occur in HIV-infected patients without prior history of psoriasis. It may be very severe.	Topical steroids, tar preparations, zidovudine, ultraviolet B light treatments
	Photosensitivity reaction is usually pruritic and hyperpigmented. May be associated with sulfa, NSIAD's, and other drugs	Discontinue offending drug. Sunscreen. Topical steroids.
Maculopapular	Molluscum contagiosum–3–5 mm flesh-colored, pearly, umbilicated lesions on face, genitals, and perianal region	Cryotherapy or electrocautery
	Kaposi's sarcoma– purple to pinkish-red, variable in size and found anywhere on skin or in mouth.	See chapter on Kaposi's sarcoma for treatment.
	Candida may cause red, pruritic macules, plaques.	Combinations of topical antifungal with mild steroids. May need systemic antifungals.

(continued)

TABLE 9–1 (continued)

Description of Lesion	Possible Causes	Treatment
	Drug eruptions are most often because of TMP/SMX. May cause urticaria, erythema multiforme.	Depending on severity of reaction, consider discontinuation of offending drug.
	Insect bites–HIV-infected patients may have severe reactions to flea, mosquito bites, and scabies.	Scabies–treat with permethrin or lindane. Mosquito, flea bites–use repellants, antihistamines, or topical steroids.
	Others: Syphilis, disseminated histoplasmosis, cryptococcus, mycobacterial infect.	See chapters on specific diseases.
Nodular, verrucous, or ulcerative lesions.	Bacillary angiomatosis-bacterial infection difficult to culture, similar to cat-scratch fever. May be confused with Kaposi's sarcoma. Diagnosis by biopsy. Appear as vascular papules, nodules, and plaques. May have fever, night sweats, and weight loss Visceral or bony involvement may occur	Erythromycin or doxycycline for 6–8 weeks or more.
	Mycobacterial infections–disseminated to skin. Fungal infections–especially histoplasmosis, coccidioidomycosis.	See chapter on *Mycobacterium*. See appropriate chapter.

(continued)

TABLE 9–1 *(continued)*

Description of Lesion	Possible Causes	Treatment
	Lymphoma–HIV associated, non-Hodgkins. May present with oral, or anorectal lesions.	See chapter on Lymphoma.
	Varicella zoster–Chronic zoster may be nodular or verrucous.	See chapter on Varicella zoster.
	Papilloma virus (especially condyloma acuminata)	For lesions small in size and few in number, consider podophyllin or cryotherapy.
		Large or numerous lesions may require surgery or laser treatment.
Vesicular or bullous lesions	Herpes simplex or varicella zoster.	See chapters on Herpes and Varicella.
	Impetigo	Systemic antistaphylococcal antibiotic
Hair and nail changes		
Hair may thin or straighten.	Unknown cause	
Eyelashes may elongate.	Unknown cause	
Yellowing of nails. Ridging of nails.	Unknown cause	
Dark pigmentation of nails.	Zidovudine	
	Fungal onychomycosis	Systemic antifungals

Diarrhea

> Possible causes include: *Salmonella, Shigella, Campylobacter, C. difficile, Giardia, Isospora,* Cryptosporidia, Microsporidia, *Mycobacterium tuberculosis* or *avium,* CMV, and malignancy

Diarrhea
↓

Laboratory studies
Blood
  Serum electrolytes—to assess need for intravenous intervention

Stool Studies
  Fecal leukocytes (rarely useful)
  Culture for *Shigella, Salmonella, Campylobacter,* and *Yersinia*
  Ova and parasites x 3 for *Giardia, Entamoeba histolytica, Cryptosporidium, Isospora belli*
  Acid fast stain and culture—for *Mycobacterium avium.* may indicate colonization or infection.
  C. difficile toxin

→ Empiric treatment directed at symptom control should begin while diagnostic workup is in progress. This treatment includes:
Dietary measures such as avoiding lactose or adding oral lactase enzyme. High calorie, low fat diet recommended.
Kaopectolin or antimotility agents such as loperamide, diphenoxylate with atropine, paregoric, or tincture of opium.
Octreotide (synthetic somatostatin) may be beneficial in some refractory cases.

↓

Definitive treatment is dependent on diagnosis (see chapters on specific causes for treatment details).

↓

If stool studies negative, consider endoscopy for small bowel or colon biopsy—may identify CMV, Kaposi's sarcoma, lymphoma, microsporidia, inflammatory bowel disease.
Empiric antibiotics such as TMP/SMX, ciprofloxacin, metronidazole, or paramomycin may be tried if no diagnosis is obtained despite complete workup.

Fatigue

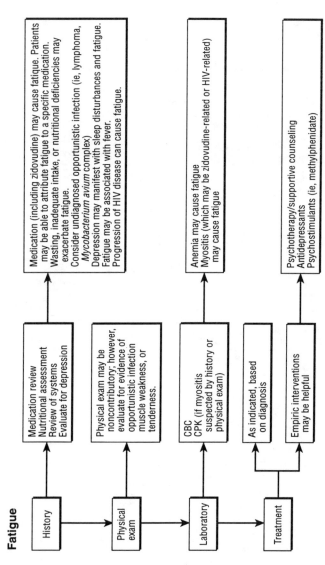

9. DIAGNOSIS OF COMMON COMPLAINTS

Fever

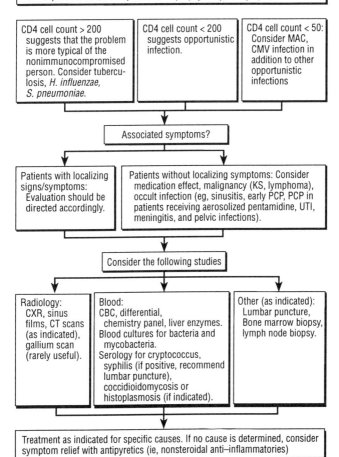

Hepatomegaly/Elevated Liver Enzymes

Possible causes include: Hepatitis A, B, or C; medication-related; MAC; lymphoma; Kaposi's sarcoma; CMV; cholangitis or papillary stenosis (especially from CMV, cryptosporidium); acalculus cholecystitis; *Cryptococcus*, coccidioidomycosis, histoplasmosis, bacillary angiomatosis.

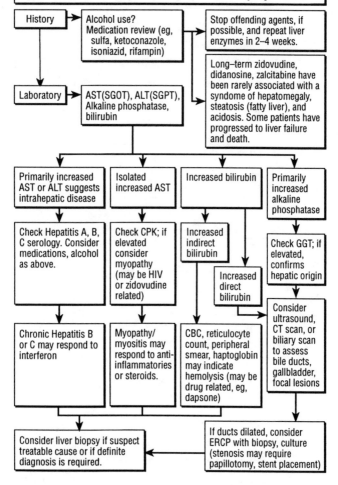

9. DIAGNOSIS OF COMMON COMPLAINTS

Headaches, Seizures, and Focal Neurologic Findings

Possible causes include: toxoplasma encephalitis, cryptococcal meningitis, progressive multifocal leukoencephalopathy (PML), neurosyphilis, lymphoma, herpes encephalitis, CMV encephalitis, HIV encephalitis, and cerebrovascular accident.

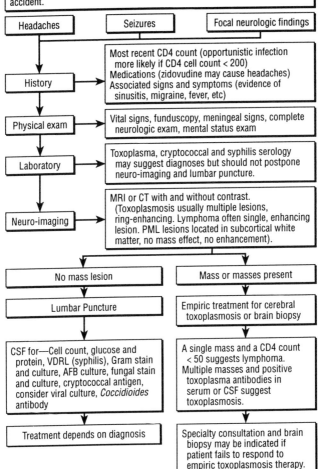

| Headaches | Seizures | Focal neurologic findings |

History → Most recent CD4 count (opportunistic infection more likely if CD4 cell count < 200). Medications (zidovudine may cause headaches). Associated signs and symptoms (evidence of sinusitis, migraine, fever, etc)

Physical exam → Vital signs, funduscopy, meningeal signs, complete neurologic exam, mental status exam

Laboratory → Toxoplasma, cryptococcal and syphilis serology may suggest diagnoses but should not postpone neuro-imaging and lumbar puncture.

Neuro-imaging → MRI or CT with and without contrast. (Toxoplasmosis usually multiple lesions, ring-enhancing. Lymphoma often single, enhancing lesion. PML lesions located in subcortical white matter, no mass effect, no enhancement).

No mass lesion
Lumbar Puncture

CSF for—Cell count, glucose and protein, VDRL (syphilis), Gram stain and culture, AFB culture, fungal stain and culture, cryptococcal antigen, consider viral culture, *Coccidioides* antibody

Treatment depends on diagnosis

Mass or masses present
Empiric treatment for cerebral toxoplasmosis or brain biopsy

A single mass and a CD4 count < 50 suggests lymphoma. Multiple masses and positive toxoplasma antibodies in serum or CSF suggest toxoplasmosis.

Specialty consultation and brain biopsy may be indicated if patient fails to respond to empiric toxoplasmosis therapy.

Odynophagia/Dysphagia

Possible causes include: *Candida*, CMV, herpes, aphthous ulceration, Kaposi's sarcoma, lymphoma, idiopathic giant esophageal ulcers.

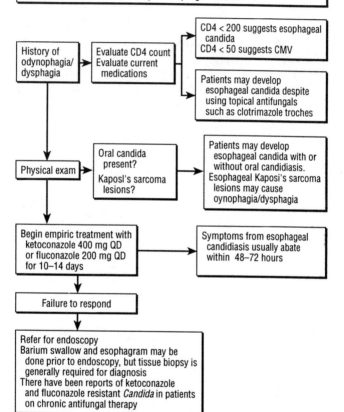

Peripheral Neuropathy

Possible causes include: predominantly sensory neuropathy (also called distal symmetric polyneuropathy), toxic neuropathy (didanosine, zalcitabine, stavudine, alcohol, INH, dapsone), B₁₂ deficiency, syphilis, hypothyroidism, diabetes mellitus, polyradiculitis, inflammatory demyelinating polyneuropathy, and vacuolar myelopathy.

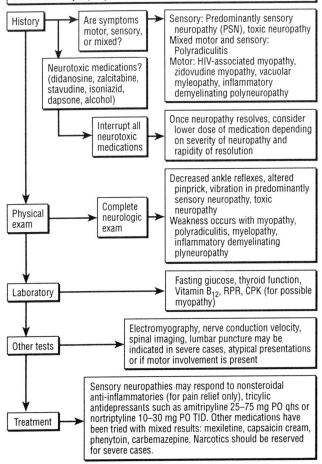

History → Are symptoms motor, sensory, or mixed? → Sensory: Predominantly sensory neuropathy (PSN), toxic neuropathy
Mixed motor and sensory: Polyradiculitis
Motor: HIV-associated myopathy, zidovudine myopathy, vacuolar myelopathy, inflammatory demyelinating polyneuropathy

Neurotoxic medications? (didanosine, zalcitabine, stavudine, isoniazid, dapsone, alcohol) → Interrupt all neurotoxic medications → Once neuropathy resolves, consider lower dose of medication depending on severity of neuropathy and rapidity of resolution

Physical exam → Complete neurologic exam → Decreased ankle reflexes, altered pinprick, vibration in predominantly sensory neuropathy, toxic neuropathy
Weakness occurs with myopathy, polyradiculitis, myelopathy, inflammatory demyelinating plyneuropathy

Laboratory → Fasting glucose, thyroid function, Vitamin B₁₂, RPR, CPK (for possible myopathy)

Other tests → Electromyography, nerve conduction velocity, spinal imaging, lumbar puncture may be indicated in severe cases, atypical presentations or if motor involvement is present

Treatment → Sensory neuropathies may respond to nonsteroidal anti-inflammatories (for pain relief only), tricylic antidepressants such as amitripyline 25–75 mg PO qhs or nortriptyline 10–30 mg PO TID. Other medications have been tried with mixed results: mexiletine, capsaicin cream, phenytoin, carbemazepine. Narcotics should be reserved for severe cases.

106 HIV/AIDS PRIMARY CARE HANDBOOK

Respiratory Complaints

Possible causes include: pneumococcus, *H. influenzae*, *Mycobacterium tuberculosis* or *avium* or *kansasii*, *Pneumocyctis carinii*, CMV, herpes, Kaposi's sarcoma, coccidioidomycosis, histoplasmosis, *Cryptococcus*, and lymphoma. Also, anemia, and congestive heart failure may cause dyspnea.

History Symptoms? Last CD4 count?
- CD4 > 200 suggest bacterial or mycobacterial infection
- CD4 < 200 suggest PCP, fungal, or other opportunistic infection

Physical exam (with attention to pulmonary and cardiovascular systems)
- Shortness of breath, fever, and dyspnea on exertion suggest PCP
- Hemoptysis suggests bacterial or mycobacterial infection or Kaposi's sarcoma

Radiology laboratory, and other studies
- Chest x-ray is essential. Lobar infiltrates suggest bacterial cause. Bilateral interstitial infiltrates suggest PCP. Tuberculosis may have atypical appearance. Adenopathy on CXR suggests Kaposis's sarcoma, MAC, or lymphoma. CT scan or gallium scan may be indicated if CXR is nondiagnostic or patient fails to respond to treatment.
- PPD and controls—may be helpful although anergy is common at low CD4 levels.
- Blood cultures—if fever present. Arterial blood gas—$PO_2 < 80$ suggests PCP, CMV. Pulse oximetry may be deceiving. Serum LDH—nonspecifically elevated in extensive pulmonary disease. Coccidioidomycosis or histoplasmosis serology if at risk.

Diagnostic procedures
- Sputum induction with hypertonic saline.
- Bronchoscopy with lavage/biopsy should be performed if sputum is negative or sooner if indicated by disease severity.
- Gram stain and culture. Acid fast bacilli stain and culture. PCP studies—cytology and direct/indirect fluorescent antibody stains (less sensitive in patients on aerosol pentamidine). Fungal stain and culture.

Treatment depends on diagnosis
- Empiric treatment may be indicated by the severity of the illness. Patients with > 200 CD4 cells should receive coverage for *H. flu.* and pneumococcus. Patients with < 200 CD4 cells should receive coverage for both bacterial pathogens and PCP. Coverage for tuberculosis should be strongly considered for all patients in areas of high TB prevalence until acid fast cultures return.

10

HIV Infection in Women

While the recommendations in this book apply to both sexes, this chapter will discuss issues specific to HIV-infected women.

Recommendations

Reproductive counseling including a discussion about contraceptive techniques is advised for HIV-infected women. Pap smears should be taken every 4 to 6 months. Colposcopy is indicated for any abnormality, ie, persistent inflammatory atypia.

Gynecologic Concerns

All women contemplate whether or not to have children. Reproductive counseling should be initiated at the first visit and continued subsequently, preferably before pregnancy occurs. The primary practitioner's role is to recognize and explore the patient's wishes and to provide information allowing the patient to make as informed a decision as possible. HIV infection is only 1 among multiple factors influencing a woman's decision on childbearing. An open, nonjudgmental discussion of the patient's personal circumstances, social and familial support system, and health status is encouraged.

Women must be informed about the following:

1. Risk of transmission of HIV to a fetus and baby
2. Impact of HIV infection and its complications (ie, toxoplasmosis, herpes simplex, etc) on the pregnancy
3. Impact of pregnancy on the course of HIV disease
4. Possible effects of HIV-related medication on the fetus and baby
5. Course of perinatally acquired pediatric HIV infection.

Contraception techniques should be discussed in detail with heterosexual or bisexual women. Information should be given on contraceptive effectiveness against pregnancy as well as against sexually transmitted diseases (Table 10–1). The effect of specific contraceptive technique on the course of HIV infection must be considered. HIV is present in vaginal secretions, and sexual partners of HIV-infected women are at risk of infection even when safer sex practices are used. When both sexual partners are HIV-infected, condoms and safer sex measures are encouraged to avoid transmission of sexually transmitted diseases (including other strains of HIV).

Gynecologic Infections

Gynecologic infections may be more severe in HIV-infected women. Treatment failures and recurrent infections frequently occur. *Candida* vaginitis may be the first sign of HIV infection. Although it occurs in women with CD4 counts above 500, symptoms often worsen with declining CD4 counts. Initial treatment with topical antifungal medications is generally attempted; treatment failures, or frequent recurrences may require oral imidazole treatment and possibly long-term suppression. Genital ulcers, such as chancroid and herpes, may take longer to resolve or be refractory to treatment in HIV-infected women. Cytomegalovirus infection has been evident on biopsies of some genital ulcers. The presence of ulcerative lesions may facilitate transmission of HIV to sexual partners.

TABLE 10-1. EFFECTIVENESS OF METHODS TO PREVENT PREGNANCY AND SEXUALLY TRANSMITTED DISEASES

Method	Estimatated Effectiveness Against STDs	Contraceptive Effectiveness		Comments
		High	Low	
Oral contraceptives	None. Decreases risk of PID	99%	96%	Unclear effects on immune system; Antibiotics may decrease efficacy.
Male condoms	30–60% (lower than expected because of misuse or nonuse).	98%	88%	Women have limited control over use
Female condoms	Not Available	Not Available	85%	Cumbersome
Diaphragm	50–75% for cervical organisms.	99%	82%	Vaginal mucosa has limited STD protection (from spermicide); Vaginal trauma may occur during insertion/removal

(continued)

TABLE 10-1. (continued)

Methods	Estimated Effectiveness Against STDs	Contraceptive Effectiveness		Comments
		High	Low	
Nonoxynol-9 impregnated sponge, jelly, foam, suppositories	50%	99%	79%	Nonoxynol-9 may be a vaginal/genital irritant in high doses or if prolonged use
Intrauterine device (IUD)	None	99%	96%	Avoid because of high risk of pelvic inflammatory disease (PID)
Levonorgestrel implant (Norplant); Medroxyprogesterone acetate (Depo-Provera)	None	99%	Not Available	There is no evidence to contraindicate use in HIV-infected women.
Tubal Ligation	None	99%	99%	

Adapted from: Rosenberg M., Gollub E. Commentary: Methods women can use that may prevent sexually transmitted disease, including HIV. *Am J Pub Health* 1992; 82:1473–8, with permission.

Pelvic inflammatory disease (PID) in HIV-infected women may manifest with more abscesses than in uninfected women and may require more extensive surgical intervention more frequently. Hospitalization and IV antibiotics are recommended for HIV-infected women with PID.

Menstrual Disorders

Amenorrhea and irregular menses (among other menstrual complaints) have been reported in HIV-infected women. With the exception of amenorrhea associated with weight loss and wasting, the cause of menstrual abnormalities in HIV infection is not well understood. Workup and management of menstrual problems should be pursued in HIV-infected women according to the patient's wishes. Many women react with discouragement and depression when menstrual disorders occur.

There is insufficient evidence to contraindicate hormonal therapy in HIV-infected women.

Cervical Dysplasia and Neoplasia

Although there are few well-controlled studies, evidence suggests that HIV-infected women are at high risk of cervical dysplasia, particularly in advanced disease (low CD4 counts) or when there is coexistent infection with human papilloma virus. At least 1 study suggests that Pap smears in HIV-infected women may not be as sensitive as in seronegative women. Colposcopy is advised if the Pap smear shows any cellular atypia (including persistent inflammation).

Invasive cervical carcinoma is now considered an AIDS defining disease in the presence of HIV infection (see Appendix for CDC Revised Classification System). There is evidence that HIV-infected women have a higher incidence of cervical neoplasia, and tend to present at a more advanced stage of disease. In 1 recent study of 16 HIV-infected women with cervical cancer, 9 of 11 deaths were due to cervical cancer, not to opportunistic infections or other complications of AIDS. In this group of 16 women, the mean CD4 count was 360. Patients with lower

CD4 counts had poorer outcomes. Treatment for HIV-infected women with cervical neoplasia should be rapid and aggressive. HIV infection is not a contraindication for surgery.

PREGNANCY IN HIV-INFECTED WOMEN

Planned and unplanned pregnancies may occur in HIV-infected women. (Reproductive counseling is discussed above.) Options regarding termination of pregnancy need to be explored in a respectful manner, taking into consideration the patient's personal, social, and physical situation.

The effect of pregnancy on the course of HIV infection appears to be minimal. Although pregnancy seems to be associated with some degree of immunosuppression in women (as manifested by declining CD4 counts), there are conflicting reports as to whether this decline is greater in HIV-infected women and what, if any, clinical implications this has.

The effect of HIV infection on pregnancy is also unclear. Many studies have reported no adverse effect on birth outcomes; some African studies, however, found increased likelihood of preterm labor, low-birth-weight, and fetal demise in HIV-infected women.

The importance of supportive services such as counselors, nutritionists, and social workers cannot be overemphasized.

Prenatal Care: Initial Visit

General prenatal guidelines apply to HIV-infected women, as do the guidelines outlined in Chapter 4 of this book. The initial visit should also include the following:

Review of Systems: Symptoms that sometimes occur during pregnancy (nausea, fatigue, weight loss, anorexia, skin lesions, abdominal pain) may be difficult to differentiate from symptoms characteristic of HIV disease progression. A high index of suspicion and careful follow-up is warranted.

Laboratory: Routine prenatal labs include: CBC, RPR, FTA, Hepatitis B surface antigen and antibody, urinalysis, rubella titer, blood type and antibody screen, alpha-fetoprotein at 15–17 weeks (with informed consent), PPD with 2 controls, Pap smear, gonorrhea culture, and chlamydia test. Toxoplasmosis titers and CMV titers are recommended as well. CD4 counts are recommended in every trimester, unless the CD4 count is > 500, in which case the second trimester measurement may be omitted.

Immunizations should be discussed on an individual basis, as limited data exist concerning risk to the fetus from most vaccines. Immunizations to be considered are outlined in Chapter 4, "Initial Visit." MMR should be withheld until postpartum.

Follow-up Visit

Frequency of Visits: Some experts recommend following patients with < 500 CD4 cells every 3 weeks until 28 weeks, then every 2 weeks until 36 weeks, then weekly until delivery. For patients with < 200 CD4 cells, some experts recommend following patients every 2 weeks until 30 weeks and then weekly. No data substantiate following patients any more frequently than the normal prenatal routine.

Laboratory: Repeating CBC, CD4 cell count, RPR, Hepatitis B surface antigen (or antibody, if Hepatitis B vaccine was given), gonorrhea culture, and chlamydia test every trimester is recommended.

Alpha-fetoprotein and Amniocentesis: These procedures need to be discussed individually with each patient. An abnormal alpha-fetoprotein is usually an indication for an amniocentesis; however, introducing a needle into the amniotic sac produces a theoretical risk of HIV transmission to the fetus. Furthermore, a targeted ultrasound may provide sufficient information to explain the abnormal alpha-fetoprotein without resorting to amniocentesis in approximately 97% of cases (O'Sullivan, 1993).

Obstetric Sonograms: There is no evidence to substantiate any benefit of routine prenatal sonograms in HIV-infected women. Some specialists recommend sonograms at 16, 28, and 36 weeks for women taking zidovudine or with CD4 counts < 200.

Antiretroviral Therapy

See Chapter 7, "Antiretroviral Therapy and Strategy" for a detailed discussion of this subject.

In February 1994, an interim review of the clinical trial ACTG 076 revealed a transmission rate of 8.3% when both mothers and their newborns received zidovudine compared to a transmission rate of 25.5% among those on placebo. ACTG 076 is a double-blind, placebo controlled study to evaluate efficacy, safety, and tolerance of zidovudine in preventing maternal-fetal HIV transmission. Zidovudine 100 mg PO 5 times daily was administered to pregnant women between 14–34 weeks of gestation. Intrapartum zidovudine was given intravenously to the women, and newborns were given zidovudine orally for the first 6 weeks of life. The zidovudine was begun within 12 hours of birth. The median CD4 count for women was 550 cells/mm^3 and their median age was 25 years. Fifty percent of the women were African-American and 29% Hispanic. The zidovudine regimen was well tolerated in the women. Although the results of ACTG 076 are directly applicable only to women who begin zidovudine between 14–34 weeks gestation, use no other antiretroviral during pregnancy, have CD4 cells > 200, and have no clinical indications for maternal antepartum zidovudine therapy, it is recommended that pregnant women with HIV infection be appraised of the study and interim results and offered zidovudine.

Prior to starting zidovudine, women should be made aware that there is no information regarding the long-term drug effects on those exposed in utero nor is there information available about the effect of discontinuing zidovudine and its effectiveness as a treatment at a later date (ie, development of resistant virus). Once zidovudine has been initiated, monitor CBC and liver function tests as indicated in Chapter 7. Zidovudine has been associated with hepatomegaly, steatosis, and elevated liver enzymes and the drug should be discontinued if these occur.

Didanosine (ddI) is being administered to some pregnant women; however, as yet, no definitive information is available. Zalcitabine (ddC) has not been studied in pregnant women, however in vitro data suggest that it has potential teratogenic effects (FDA pregnancy category C) and should therefore be discontinued during pregnancy until further information is available.

Opportunistic Infection Prophylaxis in Pregnancy

PCP prophylaxis: TMP/SMX is recommended throughout pregnancy at dosages recommended for nonpregnant adults, for those HIV-infected women with < 200 CD4 cells. Current literature does not support concerns about neonatal hyperbilirubinemia and kernicterus as a basis for withholding TMP/SMX.

Dapsone has been used in pregnant women for reasons other than PCP prophylaxis without significant problems. It should, however, be used with caution.

Pentamidine inhalation may be used, if necessary, for PCP prophylaxis.

MAC prophylaxis: Rifabutin has not been studied during pregnancy and should be avoided.

Treatment of Opportunistic Infections During Pregnancy

Opportunistic infections encountered during pregnancy can present a major problem, as many of the medications recommended for treatment are classified as FDA Pregnancy Category C. Category-C medications indicate that either animal studies demonstrate fetal risk but there are no human trials or that there are no animal or human studies available.

The possibility of acquiring an opportunistic infection during pregnancy should be discussed with every HIV-infected woman (see "General Gynecologic Concerns," above).

Intrapartum Considerations

The mode and timing of HIV transmission to the fetus is not well understood, and consequently, fetal exposure to maternal blood and vaginal secretions should be minimized. Internal scalp monitoring and scalp blood pH sampling should be avoided if possible. Avoiding operative rupture of membranes and episiotomy may also be beneficial.

Evidence suggests that cesarean section may reduce perinatal HIV transmission. Randomized trials may be needed before definitive recommendations can be made.

In order to minimize HIV exposure to the birth attendant, wall suction apparatus should be used to suction newborns. Universal precautions must be used.

Postpartum Considerations

HIV has been isolated from breast milk and breastfeeding is discouraged in the USA, where infant formula and the water supply are generally safe and readily available. More research is needed because the precise role of breastfeeding in transmitting HIV is unclear. Several studies have found a 14% increased risk of HIV transmission from mother to baby in women who breastfeed.

Contraception wishes should be addressed during prenatal care. Safer sex and the use of latex condoms must be emphasized, even in women choosing surgical sterilization or oral contraception.

REFERENCES

Bermon N: Family and reproductive issues: reproductive counseling. *AIDS Clin Care* 1993;**5**:45.

DeFerrari E et al: Midwifery care for women with human immunodeficiency virus disease in pregnancy: A demonstration project at the Johns Hopkins Hospital. *J of Nurse-Midwifery* 1993;**38**:97.

Denenberg R: *Gynecological care manual for HIV positive women.* EMIS, 1993.

Dunn DT et al: Risk of human immunodeficiency virus type 1 transmission through breastfeeding. *Lancet* 1992;**340**:585.

Heagarty M, Abrams E: Caring for HIV-infected women and children. *N Engl J Med* 1992;**326**:887.

Legg J: Women and HIV. *J Am Board of Family Practice* 1993;**6**:367.

Maiman M et al: Human immunodeficiency virus infection and invasive cervical carcinoma. *Cancer* 1993;**71**:402.

Maiman M et al: Colposcopic evaluation of human immunodeficiency virus seropositive women. *Obstet Gynecol* 1991;**78**:84.

Minkoff H, DeHovitz, J: Care of women infected with the human immunodeficiency virus. *JAMA* 1991;**266**:2253.

National Institutes of Allergy and Infectious Diseases. Clinical Alert: Important therapeutic information on the benefit of zidovudine for the prevention of transmission of HIV from mother to infant. February 22, 1994.

O'Sullivan MJ: Personal communication, December 1993.

Sperling R et al: A survey of zidovudine use in pregnant women with human immunodeficiency virus infection. *N Engl J Med* 1992;**326**:857.

Sunderland A et al: The impact of human immunodeficiency virus serostatus on reproductive decisions of women. *Obstet Gynecol* 1992;**79**:1027.

Sunderland A: Influence of human immunodeficiency virus infection on reproductive decisions. *Obstet Gynecol Clin North Am* 1990;**17**:585.

Temmerman M et al: Infection with HIV as a risk factor for adverse obstetrical outcome. *AIDS* 1990;**4**:1087.

Tovo PA: Caesarean section and perinatal HIV transmission: what next? *Lancet* 1993;**342**:630.

World Health Organization. *Consensus statement from the WHO/UNICEF consultation on HIV transmission and breastfeeding (WHO/GPA/INF/92.1).* Geneva: WHO, 1992.

11

HIV Infection in Children

The rise in the number of HIV-infected children parallels the rise in the number of HIV-infected women. Primary care practitioners may increasingly be called upon to provide infant care and screening for babies born to HIV-infected women. Perhaps the most important tasks of the primary care practitioner caring for these children are to recognize and diagnose HIV infection as early as possible and to understand that prophylactic and antiretroviral therapy may need to be initiated before reaching a definitive diagnosis of HIV infection. Providing optimal care to the at-risk child (born to an HIV-infected woman) and asymptomatic infected child requires the combined efforts of the primary care practitioner, pediatric HIV expert, nutritionist, and social worker/case manager. Symptomatic children require additional collaboration with a neurologist and neurodevelopmental specialist. Families should be appraised of available clinical trials for children.

Children acquire HIV infection through perinatal transmission (in utero, during birth, through breastfeeding) via transfusion of infected blood products (before 1985 in the USA) or from sexual abuse.

The mechanisms and timing of perinatal HIV transmission are not well understood. Factors that increase risk of perinatal infection include: maternal p24 antigenemia, low CD4 counts, placental membrane inflammation, premature birth, maternal anemia, and maternal fever. There is evidence that cesearean section has a protective effect. In addition, contracting HIV infection during pregnancy or breastfeeding is associated with a higher risk of perinatal transmission.

Zidovudine appears to lower the risk of perinatal transmission of HIV. Preliminary results of clinical trial ACTG 076 revealed that when women were given antepartum zidovudine and their newborns received zidovudine for the first 6 weeks of life, the HIV transmission rate from mother to infant was 8.3% compared with a transmission rate of 25.5% for those on placebo (see Chapter 10, "HIV Infection in Women"). The majority of children born to HIV-infected mothers will eventually lose their passively transferred maternal antibodies and become HIV-negative (and uninfected).

About 1/3 of HIV-infected children develop serious complications of AIDS within the first year of life. Median survival for HIV-infected children has improved over time, probably as a result of early diagnosis, antiretroviral therapy, and PCP prophylaxis. In one study, median survival from birth was 8 years. Forty percent of these children received zidovudine for a median of 10.3 months. There is a poorer prognosis associated with children diagnosed with PCP or encephalopathy.

Early diagnosis and therapy for HIV infection in children is of paramount importance. Pregnant women and children who are victims of sexual abuse should be offered voluntary testing for HIV.

A holistic and multidisciplinary approach to the HIV-infected child is essential (see section on "Health Maintenance" below).

When to suspect HIV infection and consider testing:

- Failure to thrive
- Recurrent serious bacterial infection
- Chronic diarrhea
- Lymphadenopathy–diffuse
- Hepatosplenomegaly
- Developmental delay or loss of attained milestones
- Recurrent or persistent oral thrush

- Maternal HIV infection or risk behaviors associated with HIV infection
- Radiographic evidence of persistent diffuse lung disease

Screening of Infants Born to Seropositive Women

The initial visit should occur between 2 weeks and 2 months of age.

History: A general history should be obtained. Inquire about father and siblings' HIV status. Current medications should be noted as well as any family history of tuberculosis.

Past Medical/Birth History: Inquire regarding maternal infections, perinatal or birth complications, birth weight, Hepatitis B, and RPR serology.

Review of Systems: Child should be assessed for appropriate weight gain, feeding history, fevers, adenopathy, skin rash, oral sores/thrush, cough, respiratory distress, diarrhea, neurologic problems.

Social History: Information about living conditions, telephone availability, community, psychological, emotional, financial resources, and employment (of parents) should be obtained. Medicaid, WIC, and other assistance obtained or needed should also be discussed with guardian, parent, or social worker/case manager.

Pretest Counseling—Expectations and Questions: Be sensitive to the fact that if a child is found to be HIV-infected, it has implications for the entire family—the mother is most likely HIV-positive and the father and siblings may also be infected.

Physical Examination: A complete physical examination is required. Height, weight, and head circumference should be recorded on growth chart. Developmental assessment should be performed at each visit.

Laboratory: The following tests should be performed at the first visit (between 2 weeks and 2 months of age):

1. CBC with differential, platelets, reticulocytes, absolute CD4 count, and percent lymphocytes CD4. These tests are used to assess need for PCP prophylaxis.
2. HIV antibody tests (to document risk).

3. HIV culture and Polymerase Chain Reaction (PCR) test and p24 antigen assay.
4. Quantitative immunoglobulins.
5. Liver function tests.

Health Maintenance

Immunizations: The following is an immunization timetable:

2 months: DTP and IPV (inactivated Salk polio vaccine) HIB*, HBV**
4 months: DTP, IPV, HIB*, HBV**
6 months: DTP, IPV (optional), HIB*, HBV**
6–12 months: Measles vaccine (in high risk areas)
12 months: MMR*** (in high risk areas if measles vaccine not given prior), PPD
15 months: MMR***, DTP, HIB*
4–6 years: DTP, IPV, MMR (second dose)

* HIB (*Haemophilus influenzae* type b vaccine)–primary series and booster series should be given according to manufacturer's instructions.

** HBV (Hepatitis B vaccine) may be given to infants born to HBsAg negative women according to 2 schedule options. See ACIP/CDC recommendations or manufacturer's instructions. In HBsAg positive women, HBV should be initiated at birth along with HBIG.

*** Measles serostatus should be monitored after immunization as IVIG is indicated after measles exposure for children who fail to mount an appropriate antibody response (see below).

We also recommend for HIV-infected children:

Pneumococcal vaccine (one dose after age 2).
Influenza vaccine (yearly after 6 months of age).
PPD yearly with control.
Passive immunization (immune globulin) after exposure to measles, varicella, or hepatitis.

Siblings and other children or adults living with HIV-infected children should receive IPV instead of OPV because of the possibility of live-virus shedding and theoretical risk of transmission to the immunocompromised host.

HIV has been isolated in breast milk. Although its role in transmission is unclear, breastfeeding is discouraged in the USA where infant formula and clean, safe water is readily available.

Comprehensive and Anticipatory Health Maintenance

Nutritional counseling is advised for all at-risk children and their families. The nutritional status of HIV-infected children should be monitored (including screening for iron-deficiency anemia) and nutritional supplementation begun promptly when indicated. Avoidance of raw eggs, raw milk, raw shellfish, or undercooked meat is advised.

Families need to learn universal precautions for handling blood and bloody secretions from HIV-infected children. There is no evidence to suggest that HIV can be transmitted through casual contact and families should be so informed. The need to seek medical advice promptly after exposure to measles, varicella, or tuberculosis should be emphasized.

Normal schooling is encouraged. Some school boards have special committees which will notify and further educate the principal and teacher regarding the child's HIV status (and the implication for education) after consent from the child's guardian has been obtained. Such notification is valuable when the child's medical condition begins to interfere with his or her schooling.

Psychosocial assessment and supportive counseling should be provided by trained personnel for the affected child and family. Social service interventions are frequently indicated. Foster care may eventually be required for many HIV-infected children.

Opportunities for enrollment in clinical trials, when feasible, should be discussed on a periodic basis.

FOLLOW-UP EXAMINATION

Interpretation of Laboratory Results

HIV Antibody Test: Because of the presence of maternal antibodies in infants up to 15–18 months of age, standard IgG ELISA and Western Blot HIV tests are not reliable indicators of infection. The test is obtained early in order to document risk so that the child may receive special social services. HIV antibody tests are repeated every 3 months during the first year of life and at 18 and 24 months or until definitive infection is confirmed. Two negative tests are recommended before informing the parent that the child is not infected (assuming the physical examination and HIV culture, p24 antigen, or PCR are negative).

A new HIV-IgA immunoblot test has been found to be quite effective in detecting HIV infection in infants 3 months and older. This test is unavailable in most localities.

HIV Culture/PCR/p24 antigen: A positive HIV culture is definitive for infection but a negative culture does not rule out infection.

PCR (polymerase chain reaction) has been found to be a sensitive test for early detection of HIV infection if performed correctly in a qualified laboratory.

The p24 antigen assay is less sensitive than HIV culture or PCR.

Using the above techniques, approximately 95% of infected infants can be identified within the first 6 months of life. A definitive diagnosis of HIV infection is made if any 2 tests are positive (including 2 different tests or the same test repeated on 2 different occasions). Virologic testing should be done soon after birth and repeated at 3–6 months of age. If results are negative, continue HIV antibody testing as previously discussed. Of course, the diagnosis of an AIDS-defining infection or condition in a child born to a seropositive mother confirms HIV infection even if virologic tests are negative.

CBC, Differential, Platelets: Anemia may occasionally result from maternal zidovudine use.

CD4 Cells: The normal range of CD4 cells is higher in

children than in adults. CD4 cell counts should be monitored every 3 months and PCP prophylaxis and antiretroviral therapy initiated accordingly even without definitive evidence of HIV infection (see below). Before initiating any therapy based on CD4 count, consider repeating the CD4 count to confirm the value.

Quantitative Immunoglobulins: Hypergammaglobulinemia is common. Hypogammaglobulinemia may occur and may be associated with false-negative HIV antibody tests.

Frequency of Follow-Up

Asymptomatic Children: These children should be followed for routine visits at 1, 2, 4, 6, 9, 12, 15, and 18 months. A careful physical examination and developmental assessment should be performed as well as immunizations and routine laboratory tests as previously outlined.

Symptomatic Children: Children with failure to thrive, chronic diarrhea, recurrent serious bacterial infections, lymphadenopathy, hepatosplenomegaly, or developmental delay should be referred to specialists for consultation. Coordination of care may be arranged between the primary practitioner and pediatric AIDS specialist.

Symptomatic children with and without CNS abnormalities need close neurologic follow-up with neurodevelopmental assessment and brain CT or MRI performed periodically to evaluate progression of disease and indicate the need for change of medical therapy.

PNEUMOCYSTIS CARINII PNEUMONIA PROPHYLAXIS

The CDC guidelines for PCP Prophylaxis are based on information regarding the early onset of PCP in children, the high mortality rate associated with PCP, and data on the CD4 counts of children with PCP.

These guidelines apply to children who meet the following criteria: (1) HIV-infected or (2) HIV seropositive or (3) Less than 12 months old and born to an HIV-infected mother, and (4) Meet age/CD4 criteria listed below.

Age/CD4 Criteria for PCP Prophylaxis

Ages 1–11 months: CD4 cell count is < 1500 (or CD4% is < 20)

Ages 12–23 months: CD4 cell count is < 750 (or CD4% is < 20)

Ages 24 months–5 years: CD4 cell count is < 500 (or CD4% is < 20)

Ages 6 years and older: CD4 cell count is < 200 (or CD4% is < 20)

Initiate PCP prophylaxis at any age for children with a previous episode of PCP.

Recommended Drug Regimen for Children Older than One Month

TMP/SMX 150 mg TMP component per m2 per day given orally in divided doses twice daily, (or in a single dose) three times per week.

Adjust dose upwards as child grows. Total daily dose should not exceed 320 mg TMP with 1600 mg SMX.

Obtain baseline CBC, differential, platelets, and liver function tests and monitor them every 4-8 weeks.

Discontinue PCP prophylaxis in those children who are determined not to be HIV-infected.

If patients are unable to tolerate TMP/SMX, consider dapsone (2 mg/kg/day–not to exceed 100 mg) or pentamidine given intravenously for infants and young children or by aerosol for older children.

Mycobacterium Avium Complex (MAC) Prophylaxis

At this time, clinical trials evaluating the safety and efficacy of rifabutin in children are underway.

ANTIRETROVIRAL AGENTS

Indications

Consider 6 weeks of zidovudine therapy for infants born to HIV-infected women who have received zidovudine during pregnancy (see zidovudine section below).

Consider antiretroviral therapy for children with AIDS defining infections or malignancies.

Antiretroviral therapy is an option for children with HIV-associated symptoms such as wasting or failure to thrive (fall from growth curve, or below 5th percentile for age, or crossing 2 percentiles over time); progressive encephalopathy; recurrent septicemia or meningitis (more than 2 episodes); thrombocytopenia ($< 75,000$ µg on 2 separate occasions); hypogammaglobulinemia (IgG < 250).

In addition, consider antiretroviral therapy for children with lymphoid interstitial pneumonitis, parotitis, splenomegaly, oral candidiasis, diarrhea (unexplained, persistent, or recurrent), HIV-related cardiomyopathy, nephrotic syndrome, or elevated liver function tests (> 5-fold normal), recurrent bacterial infections such as sinusitis or pneumonia, recurrent herpes simplex or zoster, neutropenia (< 750/µg), or anemia.

Children with CD4 cells below age-related criteria (listed below) should receive antiretroviral therapy.

< 1 year: CD4 count < 1750/ml of blood (or CD4% < 30)
1–2 years: CD4 count < 1000 (or CD4% < 25)
2–6 years: CD4 count < 750 (or CD4% < 20)
≥ 6 years: CD4 count < 500 (or CD4% <20)

Note that HIV-positive children with normal immune function and isolated lymphadenopathy, hepatomegaly, or hypergammaglobulinemia are considered asymptomatic and antiretroviral therapy is not recommended at this time.

Antiretroviral therapy should be initiated with zidovudine and changed to didanosine if there is evidence of zidovudine failure or intolerance.

Zidovudine (ZDV, Trade name—Retrovir)

This antiretroviral agent has been approved by the FDA for the use in HIV-infected children over 3 months of age, however, as previously described, it can be used in younger infants. An interim review of clinical trial ACTG 076 found a decreased risk of HIV transmission when maternal zidovudine and neonatal zidovudine were given. Zidovudine was given to infants for the first 6 weeks of life beginning within the first 12 hours after birth. The only significant side effect was mild anemia, which resolved post-therapy.

Dosage:

0–2 weeks old: 2 mg/kg/dose PO Q 6 hours.
2–4 weeks old: 3 mg/kg/dose PO Q 6 hours.
4 weeks–13 years old: 180 mg/m^2/dose PO Q 6 hours.

Toxicities: Toxicities are similar to those for adults—anemia and neutropenia.
Monitor: CBC, differential, and platelets should be assessed every 4–6 weeks, and liver function tests evaluated every 8–12 weeks.

Didanosine (ddI, Trade name—Videx)

This medication has been approved by the FDA for children over 6 months of age. Zidovudine and didanosine are the only approved antiretroviral agents for use in children.
Dosage: 90–135 mg/m^2/dose (usual dose 100 mg/m^2/dose) PO Q 12 hours. Should be taken on an empty stomach—half an hour before or after eating.
Indications: Symptomatic children should receive didanosine, when zidovudine is contraindicated, not tolerated, or when symptoms are progressing despite zidovudine.
Toxicities: The toxicity of this medication is similar to adults—pancreatitis (5% of children). Depigmentation of the retina has been observed in approximately 5% of children.

Monitor: Dilated retinal examination every 6 months or if any visual change occurs is advised.

For children with intolerance to, or disease progression in spite of zidovudine or didanosine, enrollment in clinical trials and consultation with knowlegable experts is encouraged.

OTHER THERAPIES

IV Immune Globulin (IVIG)

Some studies have found monthly doses of IVIG to reduce bacterial infections and hospitalizations in HIV-infected children. There is no evidence of prolonged survival with IVIG. Children with hypogammaglobulinemia and recurrent or chronic bacterial infections may benefit from IVIG (400 mg/kg/dose every 28 days). In addition, children who have failed to develop an antibody response to 2 MMR vaccines and who live in high-risk communities should receive IVIG. High-dose IVIG may also be indicated for children with HIV infection and thrombocytopenia unresponsive to antiretrovirals. Consultation with experts in the administration of IVIG in HIV-infected children is recommended.

COMMON PEDIATRIC HIV-ASSOCIATED INFECTIONS AND CONDITIONS

Pediatric HIV infection is a multisystem disease. Organ system involvement includes pulmonary disease (lymphoid interstitial pneumonitis—L.I.P. and PCP), cardiomyopathy, nephropathy, encephalopathy or neurologic dysfunction (in up to 50% of children), dermatologic, and hematologic abnormalities.

The most common opportunistic infections are PCP and *Candida.* Disseminated CMV, cryptosporidiosis and *Mycobacterium avium*-intracellulare infections are also common.

Pneumocytis Carinii Pneumonia

PCP is the most common opportunistic infection in children. Mortality was high in the past with median survival of 1 month in 1 study, but has been markedly decreased by early diagnosis and treatment. The estimated risk of PCP during the first year of life of a HIV-infected child is 7–20%. Median survival after diagnosis of PCP is 19 months.

Presentation: Median age of onset is 5 months of age. Symptoms are progressive with low grade fever and increased respiratory rate. Hypoxia in the presence of a mild febrile respiratory illness and often negative chest examination is a common presentation.

Diagnosis: CXR may be normal initially with progression to bilateral perihilar or interstitial infiltrates. Bronchoscopy may be required for definitive diagnosis.

Treatment: IV TMP/SMX is the drug of choice. IV pentamidine is an alternative. Adjunctive steroids may be useful.

Lymphoid Interstitial Pneumonitis

L.I.P. is the most common AIDS defining illness of HIV-infected children. L.I.P. carries a relatively better prognosis than PCP with a median survival of 72 months. Diagnosis is based on pathologic evidence, however, presumptive diagnosis is discussed below.

Presentation: Symptoms may wax and wane and include dry cough, wheezing, and respiratory distress. Bacterial superinfections are common and can present with worsened cough and fever.

Diagnosis: Presumptive diagnosis is made when CXR reveals typical bilateral reticulonodular interstitial infiltrates persisting longer than 2 months despite empiric antibiotics. Other causes of pulmonary disease must be excluded.

Treatment: There is no treatment, but steroids are used for patients with oxygen dependency. Bronchodilators are often helpful in reducing symptoms.

HIV Encephalopathy

A wide range of CNS symptoms from learning disability to severe spastic encephalopathy may be presented. Zidovudine has been shown to markedly improve some patients.

HIV Cardiomyopathy

Often begins with cardiomegaly on CXR (but normal function on echocardiogram). May progress over months to symptomatic congestive heart failure.

HIV Nephropathy

Early evidence of proteinuria with later development of bouts of nephrotic syndrome. HIV nephropathy rarely causes death.

REFERENCES

Centers for Disease Control. Hepatitis B virus: A comprehensive strategy for eliminating transmission in the United States through universal childhood vaccination: Recommendations of the Immunization Practices Advisory Committee (ACIP). *MMWR* 1991;**40 (No. RR-13)**:1.

Centers for Disease Control. Guidelines for prophylaxis against *Pneumocystis carinii* pneumonia for children infected with human immunodeficiency virus. *MMWR* 1991;**40 (No. RR-2)**:1.

Dunn DT et al: Risk of human immunodeficiency virus type 1 transmission through breastfeeding. *Lancet* 1992;**340**:585.

Grubman S, Oleske J: Primary care for the HIV-infected child. *PAACNotes* January 1993;18.

Larke RPB: HIV Infection in Children. *PAACNotes* January 1993;22.

National Institute of Allergy and Infectious Diseases. Clinical Alert: Important therapeutic information on the benefit of zidovudine for the prevention of the transmission of HIV from mother to infant. February 22, 1994.

Scott GB et al: Survival in children with perinatally acquired human immundeficiency virus type 1 infection. *N Engl J Med* 1989;1791.

Simonds RJ et al: *Pneumocystis carinii* pneumonia among US children with perinatally acquired HIV infection. *JAMA* 1993;**270:**470.

St. Louis M et al: Risk for perinatal HIV-1 transmission according to maternal immunologic, virologic, and placental factors. *JAMA* 1993;**269:**2853.

Tovo P-A: Caesarean section and perinatal HIV transmission: What next? (Commentary) *Lancet* 1993;**342:**630.

Tovo P-A: Prognostic factors and survival in children with perinatal HIV infection. *Lancet* 1992;**339:**449.

Working Group on Antiretroviral Therapy: National Pediatric HIV Resource Center. Antiretroviral therapy and medical management of the human immunodeficiency virus-infected child. *Pediatr Infect Dis J* 1993;**12:**513.

12
HIV & Nutrition

Richard S. Beach, MD, PhD, &
Cynthia A. Thomson, MS, RD, CNSD

Nutrition is an essential component in the care of HIV-infected individuals. Early in the HIV pandemic it was noted that advanced HIV infection was frequently associated with marked weight loss and severe malnutrition. Indeed, in sub-Saharan Africa, HIV-related disease was first known as "slim disease." During the past decade it has become apparent that patients at all stages of HIV-spectrum disease are at increased risk of nutritional deficiencies. In addition, nutritional disorders contribute to HIV-associated morbidity and mortality. Weight loss, cachexia, loss of lean body mass, and specific nutrient deficiencies are commonly seen in HIV-infected individuals. The cause of malnutrition is thought to be multifactorial and related to loss of appetite, malabsorption, increased losses (vomiting, diarrhea, renal losses, etc), and alterations in metabolism.

Any HIV-infected person should be considered at risk for malnutrition. It is estimated that some 97% of HIV-positive patients experience substantial weight loss prior to death. Moreover, the degree of body weight loss predicts mortality, for example, when actual body weight approaches 60% of ideal body weight, death is very likely to occur even in the absence of specific underlying diseases. Other markers of overall nutritional status such as measures of lean body mass (midarm muscle circumference, bioelectrical impedance analysis) and visceral protein status (albumin, transferrin, and prealbumin) also correlate with increased risk of mortality.

Importantly, wasting and weight loss need not be an inevitable consequence of HIV infection. Absence of wasting and weight loss correlates with clinical stability, which may be maintained for long periods of time.

There are 2 generally distinct patterns of weight loss that tend to occur in individuals with HIV infection. Some patients present with a fairly rapid onset of progressive weight loss. These patients generally have an undiagnosed opportunistic infection. Weight loss, fatigue, anorexia, and low grade fevers may be the early nonspecific signs of it. By not monitoring body weight closely, clinicians may miss an opportunity for early detection of opportunistic infections. As long as infections remain untreated, nutritional support regimens will meet with limited success.

A second pattern of weight loss is more gradual (1–2 lbs lost every 1–2 months) and the causes are not fully understood. It is likely multifactorial as indicated above. The best treatment is prevention, much as prophylaxis is offered against various opportunistic infections. Nutritional prophylaxis requires not only increased consumption of calories and other nutrients, but also touches on aspects of lifestyle including exercise, smoking, alcohol consumption, recreational drug use, and general stress reduction. As an understanding of this form of weight loss and wasting grows, so will the therapeutic modalities available.

It should be noted that HIV-infected women are at increased risk of wasting. Wasting syndrome is the second most common AIDS-defining diagnosis among women as compared to the ninth most common AIDS-defining diagnosis in men. The reasons for this are not understood at this time.

While nutritional support is a key component of the treatment plan of HIV-infected individuals, there are certain groups of patients who need special attention. Referral to a practitioner specializing in nutritional concerns such as a clinical nutritionist or dietician is recommended (Table 12–1).

COMPONENTS OF NUTRITIONAL CARE

Nutritional Status Assessment

Diet History Analysis: At a minimum, the physician should ask for a 24-hour dietary recall. Nutritionists also include a food frequency questionnaire as well as diet records for 3 nonconsecutive days including 1 weekend day. This is useful in assessing nutritional adequacy by identifying potentially deficient nutrients. This should be performed yearly in all HIV-infected individuals and should be repeated with changes in clinical status or with significant changes in the treatment regimen.

Body composition analysis and anthropometrics: Nutritionists often perform anthropometric measurements of tricep skinfold thickness and subscapular skinfold thickness. Calipers to perform such measurements are relatively inexpen-

TABLE 12–1. INDICATIONS FOR NUTRITION REFERRAL

- Persistent complaints of nausea, emesis, diarrhea, malabsorption, or dysphagia
- Persistent oral candidiasis (thrush), oral Kaposi's sarcoma, severe oral hairy leukoplakia
- Use of herbals, megadoses of vitamins/minerals, alternative nutritional therapies
- Food access difficulties (economic, physical, etc.)
- Albumin < 3.6 mg/dl or cholesterol < 120 mg/dl
- Patients being considered for oral, enteral, or parenteral nutrition support
 Anorexia, loss of appetite secondary to any of the complications of HIV infection
 Weight loss of > 10 lbs. or >5% of usual body weight in past 3 months
 Pregnancy

sive and ancillary personnel can be trained in their use. Serial measurements are useful in evaluating changes in subcutaneous fat or somatic protein mass in patients whose weight may remain normal. A recent innovation is bioelectrical impedance analysis, which permits noninvasive testing of fat stores as opposed to lean muscle mass. These instruments have been employed in the setting of HIV infection. Serial measurements provide the most useful clinical information.

It is essential to obtain a baseline height on the patient as well as weight measurements at every clinic visit.

Evaluation of nutritional biochemical parameters: Recommended baseline data (fasting).–Albumin, prealbumin (especially if the patient has renal or hepatic disease as albumin is then not as reflective of current nutritional state), cholesterol, triglycerides, renal panel, liver enzymes, hemoglobin, serum iron, magnesium, folate, B_{12}, and serum retinol (vitamin A) with retinol binding protein are all useful, especially in a new, symptomatic patient. Some of these values will be altered by various HIV-related therapeutics.

The above data are key indicators of visceral protein or specific nutrient status and have been advised for evaluation based on current literature. Measurements of cholesterol, albumin and serum retinol may predict morbidity and mortality in HIV-infected individuals. Patients with specific symptoms or nutritional risk factors, such as alcohol abuse, may need further biochemical tests to assess specific nutritional parameters that may contribute to the disease process.

Traditional measures such as MCV and MCH tend not to be helpful as many of the medications used in HIV-infected patients alter these parameters. Ferritin is elevated in HIV infection as an acute phase reactant and is therefore not useful to assess iron stores. Measurements of some specific nutrient levels (ie, zinc and copper) may be difficult to interpret because changes in metabolism may not alter total body stores, but may promote a redistribution of these trace elements. Nonetheless, low blood levels in the face of inadequate dietary intake most likely implies a specific nutrient deficiency.

Importance of Nutrition Education

Nutritional evaluation is most effective when provided in conjunction with appropriate nutritional education. Encounters between primary practitioners and patients should encourage openness regarding the patient's nutritional (and other adjunctive treatment) practices in order to appropriately assess potentially deficient as well as overly aggressive/harmful nutritional practices. Individuals with HIV infection often feel relatively powerless in the face of their infection and their involvement in nutritional education and the beneficial aspects of nutritional follow-up (serial measurements of progress in terms of lean body mass, etc.) may serve as a significant psychological empowerment tool. It may also help to get patients more involved in all aspects of their care.

NUTRIENT SUPPLEMENTATION/AUGMENTATION

A significant percentage of HIV-infected patients will present with nutritional deficiencies despite what appears to be normal weight status and reported adequate intake. Deficiencies in vitamin B_{12}, B_6, A, E, zinc, and copper have frequently been reported and cited in the literature. Therefore, there is growing evidence that routine vitamin and mineral supplementation is warranted in this patient population to replenish depleted stores, to prevent further deficits, and to maintain optimal immune function, cognitive function, and quality of life (ie, nutrient deficiencies may be a contributing factor to the fatigue so commonly found in HIV-infected patients).

Recommended Supplementation

Clinical studies of nutrient deficiency and supplementation in HIV-infected individuals are ongoing and direct causal relationships are still unclear. Precise recommendations and exact doses of supplements are difficult to delineate. Following are some guidelines that may prove helpful.

Patients should be instructed to consume one multivitamin with mineral tablet once or twice daily with a meal. The selected supplement should contain about 200% of the RDAs for all nutrients, including zinc, selenium, and copper.

Vitamins: Monthly IM B_{12} injections or twice weekly intranasal preparations will be necessary in approximately 30% of patients who will have documented deficiency. Deficiencies of vitamin B_{12} have been associated with decreased cognitive function. B_6 deficiency has been associated with lower CD4 cells; these levels have improved with the replacement of B_6. Vitamin A (retinol) deficiency has been found to have a significant correlation with mortality and clinical instability, but caution should be exercised to avoid excess supplementation because of toxicity.

Minerals: As previously mentioned, lab measurements of nutrients may be difficult to interpret. Zinc deficiency is relatively common in HIV infection and tends to be associated with more rapid progression to AIDS. Whether this is a direct causal relationship, however, remains unclear. When supplementing zinc, use no more than 50 mg/day because higher doses are immunosuppressive. Copper and selenium deficiencies have also been seen. Iron supplementation should not be prescribed unless iron deficiency has been clearly diagnosed. Excess iron has been associated with increased risk of bacterial infection.

Antioxidants: Beta-carotene, selenium, vitamin E, vitamin C, coenzyme Q-10, and glutathione are all considered to be antioxidants, which theoretically reduce the levels of free radicals and their associated oxidative damages to tissue. They are being promoted not only for HIV-infected patients, but for patients at risk for heart disease and cancer as well. Vitamin C may be taken up to 1 gram daily. Higher doses of Vitamin C often cause gastrointestinal symptoms so doses should be started low and increased gradually. Beta-carotene in doses of 180 mg PO QD has been shown to increase CD4 counts and may also lead to increased levels of Vitamin A in patients. Coenzyme Q-10 and NAC (N-acetyl-Cysteine) have significant gastrointestinal side effects and this limits usefulness. Glutathione in its current form does not appear to be effective in reaching target cells; however, new formulations (ie, procysteine) are being explored.

Clinicians should keep in mind that the current RDAs have been established for the healthy USA population and are likely inadequate for patients with HIV, especially in the advanced stages of the disease. On the other hand, excessive supplementation can impair immunological function and caution should be taken to avoid megadose levels of supplementation. In addition, excessive doses of single nutrients have also been shown to interfere with the availability of other nutrients. For example, excess vitamin C intake will interfere with vitamin B_{12} absorption and high zinc intake blocks copper absorption.

Appetite stimulants: Appetite stimulants should be used only when other potential causes of anorexia have been addressed. Agents commonly prescribed include dronabinol (Marinol), megestrol (Megace), and cyprohepatadine (Periactin). Dronabinol results in increased appetite, weight gain, and elevated mood about 4–6 weeks after initiation of treatment. Side effects eventually cause about 1/2 of patients taking the drug to stop. Megestrol is also effective in increasing appetite though weight gain appears to be primarily fat. Side effects include impotence and diabetes mellitus. Finally, cyproheptadine has largely been used in children and its impact on appetite and weight gain is largely unknown.

Anabolic agents: Supplementation with anabolic agents may involve replacement of an endocrine factor that is present in subnormal levels (ie, testosterone) or augmenting normal hormone levels (ie, growth hormone). Studies consistently reveal that many HIV-infected men have lower than expected testosterone levels. It is unclear whether supplementation normalizes metabolism and leads to an improved ability to add lean body mass. Recent studies show that recombinant growth hormone supplementation at 0.1 mg/kg/day results in a positive nitrogen balance and deposition of new lean body mass. Use of adjunctive anabolic steroids in both parenteral (decadurabolin) and oral (oxandrolone) forms are currently in clinical trials. Some patients with HIV infection obtain these agents outside of protocols. It appears that these steroids are most effective when used in conjunction with a regular and varied exercise program.

COMMON DISEASE-RELATED COMPLICATIONS AND NUTRITIONAL ISSUES

Anorexia

Reviewing a patient's appetite provides a key piece of clinical information and should be done at every visit. Investigating the causes of inappetence is important. Potential factors include undiagnosed/untreated opportunistic infections. Medications used in HIV infection frequently have side effects that include nausea and anorexia. As the list of medication grows, the impact on the patient's overall well-being, including nutritional status must continually be reassessed. Advise small, frequent meals and calorically dense foods and beverages. Encourage shared meals and change in eating place. Supplements are indicated, and patients can learn to prepare their own high calorie/high nutrient drinks at a significantly reduced cost.

Diarrhea

It is vital to identify and treat the cause of diarrhea. Diarrhea results in increased losses of water soluble vitamins, fluids, magnesium, and zinc. Nutrient supplementation should attempt to match nutrient losses. Water soluble vitamin needs can generally be met with an additional B complex vitamin with vitamin C daily (in addition to the multivitamin-mineral supplement). Some B complex with vitamin C have excessive levels of nutrients; therefore, the patient should be advised to use a supplement that is between 100–200% of the RDAs. Fluid replacement should match fluid losses.

Lactose intolerance is likely in patients with diarrhea. In an effort to continue dairy products, which are a significant source of protein, calories, and nutrients, patients should be advised to use lactose-free dairy products or use commercial lactase preparation before meals containing milk or dairy products. High osmolality may also contribute to intolerance.

The BRATT diet (bananas, rice, applesauce, toast, and tea), used historically for children with diarrhea, has limited efficacy in the HIV population. Instituting this restricted diet will lead to significant undernutrition if used for longer than 48–72 hours. Patients should continue eating despite diarrhea.

Dysphagia

Patients with dysphagia should receive a soft diet. If the condition is severe, the risk of aspiration can increase with the consumption of thin liquids, therefore thick liquids will need to be substituted. Calorically dense supplements can be prescribed. A speech therapist's evaluation of the patient's swallowing mechanism can be helpful.

Dyspnea

Small, frequent meals are recommended. Fatigue may limit caloric consumption and assistance with feeding may be necessary. Higher fat, lower carbohydrate diet may help. Provide meals in semi-reclining position to optimize oxygen flow throughout the lungs.

Fat Malabsorption

Fat malabsorption has been diagnosed in HIV patients using the 72-hour fecal fat test. To obtain reliable results, the patient should consume a high fat (> 80 gms) diet for 2 days prior to the stool collection. If the test is positive, the patient will need instruction on a low fat diet, supplemental fat soluble vitamins, and Medium Chain Triglyceride oil.

Fever

The major nutritional concern with fever is the increased caloric expenditure and fluid losses. For each degree centigrade increase in temperature, basal caloric requirements increase by 13%, and fluid requirements will rise by 300 ml daily.

Nausea

Small, frequent meals are recommended. Cold foods may be better tolerated than warm. Avoid offending smells that may trigger nausea. It is advisable to drink fluids between meals rather than with meals.

Psychologic Stress and Depression

Psychologic disorders such as depression (especially when combined with fatigue, sleep disorders, and sexual dysfunction) commonly lead to poor or inappropriate nutritional intake. Intervention in the form of psychotherapy, support groups, and antidepressant medication is warranted.

Weight Loss

Determine the cause when possible. Consider undiagnosed opportunistic infections. In the event of an opportunistic infection, nutritional intervention should occur early. For example, early initiation of enteral feeds by nasojejunal tube feeding when the patient is unable to eat, may prevent the 10–20 lbs weight loss that often accompanies serious illness.

In the absence of, or during treatment of opportunistic infection, consider referral to a clinical nutritionist. Encourage small, frequent, calorically dense meals. Arrange assistance with meals as indicated (local programs, family, and friends) and recommend high calorie, high protein supplements such as Instant Breakfasts or a lactose-free alternative.

SPECIALIZED NUTRITION SUPPORT

Certain patients will require more aggressive nutritional support, including enteral and parenteral nutrition, to meet their nutritional needs. Table 12–2 summarizes the current indications for enteral and parenteral nutrition in HIV. **It is important to use the gut if at all possible!** There is clear evidence that enteral feeding not only maintains gut integrity, but it reduces the translocation of gut bacteria into the lymphatics and has been shown to replenish both lean and fat mass, a characteristic not shared by patients supported with TPN alone.

TABLE 12–2. INDICATIONS FOR ENTERAL AND PARENTERAL NUTRITION IN HIV PATIENTS

Enteral	Parenteral
Significant malnutrition	Intolerance to enteral feeding (half of patients will respond to refeeding with an elemental oral formula)
Partial or upper GI tract obstruction	
Severe dysphagia or esophagitis	Bowel obstruction
Severe dementia	Severe or frequently recurrent pancreatitis
Coma	
Malnutrition with inadequate oral intake	Copious/high volume diarrhea (after treatable causes have been ruled out and offending dietary components, ie, lactose, high magnesium levels, and high osmolality have been eliminated)
Prolonged intake (> 14 days) of < 50% energy needs	
Distal, lower output enterocutaneous fistulas	
Patients undergoing cancer therapies with resulting weight loss	
Supplement (nocturnal feeding) po intake	Intractable emesis
Opportunistic infection accompanied by inability to eat	High output enterocutaneous fistula
Radiation enteritis may be prevented with elemental formulas	

Patients who require specialized nutrition support should be encouraged to use the enteral route whenever possible. Cost of a supplement does not guarantee effectiveness.

Any patient requiring specialized support should be evaluated by a nutrition support team with experience in home support. Evaluation of the patient and family, in terms of ability to learn and comply with feeding regimes, is critical to this process. Improper administration of specialized nutrition support can be life-threatening. In addition, the nutrition support team will provide ongoing monitoring, which is essential to optimal care and nutritional repletion.

REFERENCES

Baum MK et al: Association of vitamin B_6 status with parameters of immune function in early HIV-1 infection. *J AIDS* 1991;**4:**1122.

Baum MK et al: Influence of HIV infection on vitamin status and requirements. *Ann NY Acad Sci* 1992;**587:**165.

Beach RS et al: Plasma vitamin B_{12} level as a cofactor in studies of human immunodeficiency virus type-1 related cognitive changes. *Arch Neurol* 1992;**49:**501.

Beach RS et al: Specific nutrient abnormalities in asymptomatic HIV infection. *AIDS* 1992;**6:**701.

Chelbowski RT et al: Nutritional status, gastrointestinal dysfunction, and survival in patients with AIDS. *Am J Gastroenterol* 1989;**84:**1288.

Guenter P et al: Relationships among nutritional status, disease progression, and survival in HIV infection. *J Acq Imm Def Syndr* 1993;**6:**1130.

Grunfeld C, Feingold K: Metabolic disturbances and wasting in the acquired immunodeficiency syndrome. *N Engl J Med* 1992;**327:**329.

Hellerstein MK et al: Current approach to the treatment of human immunodeficiency virus-associated weight loss: Pathophysiologic considerations and emerging management strategies. *Semin Oncol* 1990;**17:**17.

Keusch GT, Farthing JG: Nutritional aspects of AIDS. *AA Rev Nutr* 1990;**10:**475.

Kotler DP, Mang J, Pierson RN: Body composition analysis in patients with the acquired immunodeficiency syndrome. *Am J Clin Nutr* 1985;**42:**1255.

Kotler DP et al: Preservation of short term energy balance in clinically stable patients with AIDS. *Am J Clin Nutr* 1990;**51:**7.

Kotler DP et al: Effect of enteral alimentation upon body cell mass in patients with the acquired immunodeficiency syndrome. *Am J Clin Nutr* 1991;**53:**149.

Kotler DP et al: Magnitude of body cell mass depletion and the timing of wasting from death in AIDS. *Am J Clin Nutr* 1989;**50:**444.

Kushner RF: Bioelectrical impedance analysis: A review of principles and applications. *J Am Coll Nutr* 1992;**11:**199.

Macallan DC et al: Prospective analysis of patterns of weight change in stage IV human immunodeficiency virus infection. *Am J Clin Nutr* 1993;**58:**417.

Ott M et al: Early changes of body composition in human immunodeficiency virus-infected patients: Tetrapolar body impedance analysis indicates significant malnutrition. *Am J Clin Nutr* 1993;**57:**15.

Raiten DJ: Nutrition and HIV infection: A review of the extant knowledge of the relationship between nutrition and HIV infection. *Nutr Clin Pract* 1991;**6(Suppl 1):**15S.

Semba RD et al: Increased mortality associated with vitamin A deficiency during human immunodeficiency type 1 infection. *Arch Intern Med* 1993;**153:**2149.

Serwadda D et al: Slim disease: New disease in Uganda and its association with HTLV-III infection. *Lancet* 1985;**2:**849.

Staal FJT et al: Glutathione deficiency and human immunodeficiency virus infection. *Lancet* 1992;**339:**909.

13
Experimental & Nontraditional Treatments for AIDS

As the death toll from AIDS continues to climb, researchers work toward a more complete understanding of the human immunodeficiency virus and potential ways to alter its natural course. Numerous clinical trials involve drugs in all phases of testing and include antiretroviral, immunomodulating and antibiotic agents.

Individuals may become involved in clinical trials through academic medical centers participating in the National Institute of Allergy and Infectious Diseases (NIAID) AIDS Clinical Trials Group (ACTG) or through Community Programs for Clinical Research on AIDS (CPCRA) sponsored by the NIAID. In addition, various pharmaceutical companies have developed expanded access programs for experimental medications for HIV-infected and AIDS patients. Pharmaceutical companies also sponsor clinical trials through academic institutions, private centers, and community research initiatives.

In response to the AIDS crisis and at the urging of AIDS activist groups, the FDA has allowed an unprecedented "fast-tracking" of new drug development and approval.

Alternative and nontraditional medical practices, including the use of acupuncture, herbal medicines, megavitamins, imagery, massage, and folk remedies, to name a few, are widely used by the American population in general. A recent national survey estimated that in 1990, 425 million visits were made to providers of nontraditional therapy compared with 388 million visits to mainstream primary care practitioners.

Another survey conducted among patients at an AIDS clinic found that many used unorthodox treatments, particularly patients with higher educational levels and those with more advanced stages of disease.

Experimental and unlicensed drugs are also being used by HIV-infected individuals. Motivations include a sense that for people with AIDS, time is running out and given the limited offerings of mainstream medicine it is worth exploring unproven therapies. These therapies include:

1. Approved drugs used for off-label purposes, often with uncommon dosages, ie, acyclovir, ranitidine, cimetidine, disulfiram, levamisole, naltrexone, and pentoxifylline.
2. Drugs not approved in the USA but available elsewhere, ie, albendazole, isoprinosine, oral amphotericin B, oral N-acetylcysteine, oral ribavirin, and tinidazole.
3. Experimental drugs and therapies that are not approved anywhere, ie, tricosanthin (Compound Q), peptide-T, ozone therapy, and oral interferon.
4. Herbal and over-the-counter preparations, ie, beta-carotene, hypericin (St. John's wort), Sho-saiko-to (SSKT), and megavitamins.

The above mentioned examples are used for a variety of purposes including immune-stimulation, antiviral properties, anti-infectives or symptom relief. Some of them are currently undergoing investigation in clinical trials.

There are numerous buyers' clubs for AIDS drugs throughout the country where medications such as those previously referenced may be obtained (see "Resources for Practitioners and Patients" in the Appendix for information on selected buyers' clubs). Both approved and unapproved medications are generally imported from other countries where they are less expensive. The FDA acknowledges the presence of, and tolerates the use of buyers' clubs provided that they avoid commercialization, insure the safety of their products, and sell the drugs to individuals only for their own personal use. The FDA expects that the individuals purchasing these drugs will use them under a physician's care. The majority of buyer's clubs are nonprofit organizations. In 1992, representatives of 11 buyer's clubs developed a set of ethical principles to guide their operations. Virtually all buyer's clubs require a physician's prescription before dispensing prescription medications.

Becoming informed about available clinical trials, alternative therapies, and maintaining an open communication with patients about these issues is encouraged for practitioners caring for HIV-infected individuals. Serious drug interactions and toxicities may occur with both approved and unconventional agents, and practitioners should be apprised of the risks involved with the therapies used by their patients. Practitioners may also play a role as the patient's advocate, in helping to assess potential therapies. Their role may extend to preventing the occasional episode of gross exploitation and fraud, a situation which sometimes arises when vulnerable, often desperate people fall prey to outrageous claims.

REFERENCES

Braun J et al: A guide to underground AIDS therapies. *Patient Care* 1993:**53**.

Eisenberg D et al: Unconventional medicine in the United States: Prevalence, costs and patterns of care. *N Engl J Med* 1993;**328:**246.

Greenblatt RM et al: Polypharmacy among patients attending an AIDS clinic: Utilization of prescribed, unorthodox, and investigational treatments. *J Acquir Immune Defic Syndr* 1991;**4:**136.

14

Health Care Workers & HIV

HEALTH CARE WORKERS AND OCCUPATIONAL EXPOSURE TO HIV

Virtually all health care workers who work with HIV-infected are concerned at times about the possibility of contracting HIV from their patients. The Centers for Disease Control and Prevention, in collaboration with local and state health departments, conduct surveillance for HIV-infected health care workers as well as those diagnosed with AIDS. Follow-up investigations are undertaken to determine whether infection occurred through occupational exposure and to identify the circumstances that resulted in transmission.

Through September 1993, 39 health care workers have been reported with documented occupationally-acquired HIV infection (ie, a negative HIV-antibody tests at the time of exposure and subsequent conversion). Another 81 health care workers have possible occupationally acquired HIV infection (ie, those with past occupational exposure to HIV and without behavioral or transfusion risks, but who lack documented seroconversion as a result of the occupational exposure). The number of health care workers with occupationally acquired HIV infection is undoubtedly higher than listed because not all health care workers are evaluated for HIV infection after exposure nor are all occupationally acquired cases reported to the CDC.

Clinical laboratory technicians, nurses, and nonsurgical physicians comprise the groups with the highest number of both documented and possible occupationally acquired HIV infection. The majority of exposures were percutaneous exposures to HIV-infected blood. Of those with documented occupationally acquired HIV infection, however, 4 individuals (10% of the total) report mucocutaneous exposure only.

Several studies have found the risk of HIV transmission after percutaneous exposure to HIV-infected blood to be about 0.3–0.4%. The risk of HIV transmission after mucous membrane or cutaneous exposure is even less.

UNIVERSAL PRECAUTIONS

Because every patient and every health care worker is potentially HIV-infected, care should be taken to protect oneself and protect the patient. The CDC's recommendations for prevention of HIV transmission in health care settings should be applied universally to protect patients and health care workers.

The recommendations include:

Wear gloves when touching blood, body fluids, mucous membranes, or non-intact skin of all patients.
Wear gloves when handling items soiled with blood or body fluids.
Wear gloves when performing venipuncture or invasive procedures.
Change gloves between each patient.
Wear masks and protective eyewear or face shields when doing procedures likely to generate droplets of blood or body fluids.
Wear gowns or aprons when doing invasive procedures.
Wash hands and skin immediately and thoroughly after contact with blood and body fluids.
Do not recap needles or bend them or manipulate them in any way.

Dispose of sharp objects in puncture-resistant containers.

Although saliva is not known to transmit HIV, mouth-to-mouth resuscitation should be avoided. Resuscitation bags, mouthpieces, or other ventilation devices should be available when appropriate.

Health care workers with weeping or exudative lesions should avoid direct patient contact until the condition resolves.

Pregnant health care workers should be especially aware of the above precautions and strictly adhere to them.

Body fluids considered to be infectious include:

- Blood
- Tissues
- Cerebrospinal fluid
- Synovial fluid
- Peritoneal fluid
- Pleural fluid
- Pericardial fluid
- Amniotic fluid
- Semen
- Vaginal secretions

Universal precautions do not apply to body fluids that are not considered to be infectious, for instance, feces, nasal secretions, sputum, sweat, tears, urine, vomitus, and saliva (unless contaminated with blood). Good hygiene, however, is recommended.

While studies have documented that universal precautions are effective in reducing the health care worker's risk of exposure to HIV, there is ample evidence that universal precautions are not being routinely applied in health care settings.

POST-EXPOSURE ZIDOVUDINE IN HEALTH CARE WORKERS

When exposure to high-risk or known HIV-infected blood or body fluids occurs, what should be done? For years some medical facilities have offered zidovudine prophylaxis to health care workers with high-risk exposures. Yet despite post-exposure zidovudine prophylaxis, there have been reports that at least 8 health care workers have subsequently seroconverted.

At this time, it is impossible to ascertain whether post-exposure zidovudine (or any other antiretroviral agent) offers protection from HIV infection. To assess the efficacy of post-exposure zidovudine, a large, controlled randomized trial or longitudinal study should be implemented. A randomized trial was initiated in 1987, but it closed shortly afterwards because of failure to enroll enough participants. In view of the 8 or more health care workers who failed zidovudine prophylaxis, it is clear "that if zidovudine is protective, any protection is not absolute" (Tokars, 1993).

Various protocols for post-exposure zidovudine exist. Consensus holds that the sooner the zidovudine is initiated, the better—preferably within the first hour or so of exposure.

Recommendations include:

- Zidovudine 200 mg PO TID for 4–6 weeks *or*
- Zidovudine 200 mg PO every 4 hours for the first 3 days and then every 4 hours 5 times daily (omitting the nighttime dose) for a total of 28 days

Although the risk of HIV infection following percutaneous exposure is low, and despite the lack of data to support the use of zidovudine, every health care worker should consider requesting post-exposure zidovudine in the event an exposure occurs. Potential benefits include the possibility that HIV infection might be prevented. On a negative note, some 75% of workers taking post-exposure zidovudine reported adverse effects—most commonly nausea, fatigue, and headache. Thirty-one percent of workers actually interrupted zidovudine because of adverse reactions. Furthermore, frequent laboratory monitoring is necessary while zidovudine is being used.

For information about the CDC voluntary surveillance project for health care workers with occupational HIV exposure contact:

Hospital Infections Program
National Center for Infectious Diseases
Centers for Disease Control and Prevention

Mail Stop A-07
Atlanta, GA 30333
(404) 639-1547

HIV-INFECTED HEALTH CARE WORKERS

Despite the public outcry arising from the tragic case of a Florida dentist who possibly transmitted HIV to 6 of his patients, the risk of acquiring HIV from an infected health care worker is small—less than the risk of dying as a result of general anesthesia during surgery. The case of the Florida dentist remains the only potential documented instance of transmission of HIV to patients in a health care setting in the USA. Numerous "look back" studies have failed to find other cases related to infected surgeons or dentists.

The CDC presented recommendations on preventing HIV transmission to patients in July 1991. Although these recommendations were regarded as controversial, the CDC has yet to publish revised recommendations.

The question of whether to devise special mechanisms for dealing with HIV-infected health care workers (and if so, how) remains an issue riddled with ethical dilemmas and concerns about potential discrimination. Two points from the CDC's July 1991 recommendations bear mentioning: First, is the reiteration of the importance of Universal Precautions to protect both health care worker and patient; second is the implied recommendation that health care workers should be tested for HIV antibody and then act appropriately in accordance with their patients best interests.

REFERENCES

Centers for Disease Control. Recommendations for prevention of HIV transmission in health care settings. *MMWR* 1987;**369**(Suppl 2S):3S.

Centers for Disease Control. Recommendations for preventing transmission of human immunodeficiency virus and hepatitis B to patients during exposure-prone invasive procedures. *MMWR* 1991;**40**:1.

Centers for Disease Control. Surveillance for occupationally-acquired HIV infection. *MMWR* 1992;**41**:823.

Centers for Disease Control. Update: transmission of HIV infection during an invasive dental procedure–Florida. *MMWR* 1991;**40:**21.

Centers for Disease Control and Prevention. HIV/AIDS surveillance report. 1993;**5 (No. 3):**1.

Henderson DK et al: Risk for occupational transmission of human immunodeficiency virus type 1 (HIV-1) associated with clinical exposures: A prospective evaluation. *Ann Intern Med* 1990;**113:**740.

Lo B, Steinbrook R: Health care workers infected with the human immunodeficiency virus: the next steps. *JAMA* 1992;**267:**1100.

Marcus R, CDC Cooperative Needlestick Surveillance Group: Occupational risk of the acquired immunodeficiency syndrome among health care workers. *N Engl J Med* 1988;**319:**1118.

O'Neill TM, Abbott AV, Radecki SL: Risk of needlesticks and occupational exposure among residents and medical students. *Arch Intern Med* 1992;**152:**1451.

Tokars JI et al: Surveillance of HIV infection and zidovudine use after occupational exposure to HIV-infected blood. *Ann Intern Med* 1993;**118:**913.

Wong ES et al: Are universal precautions effective in reducing the number of occupational exposures among health care workers? *JAMA* 1991;**265:**1123.

15

Medications Commonly Used in HIV-Infected Individuals

Cindy M. Maggio, PharmD,
Kimberley J. Campbell, PharmD, RPh,
Mary Greene Manning, PharmD,
Michael D. Katz, PharmD, Teresa C. Nord,
PharmD, & Kari A. Wieland, PharmD

The following section includes a brief summary of some medications commonly used in HIV-infected people. The intent is to provide information about medications that are unfamiliar or applied in unique ways in HIV infection. This information is not intended to substitute for more detailed references, and the review of more detailed sources when using a medication for the first time or to evaluate complaints that may be related to medications is encouraged. Much of the information was extracted from primary sources such as journal articles and from various secondary sources such as the *1993 Updated Facts and Comparisons, 1993 Guide to Antimicrobial Therapy, 1993 Guide to HIV/AIDS Therapy,* and the *1993 American Hospital*

Formulary Service. Some information applicable to HIV-infected women was extracted from *Gynecological Care Manual for HIV Positive Women.* Cost information was retrieved from the *1993 Redbook,* which provides average wholesale price (AWP). Prices cited are for generic products wherever available. See Appendix for medications with payment assistance program and expanded access programs offered by pharmaceutical companies.

Note: Not all indications are FDA approved but may represent the standard of practice based on literature evaluation and community standards. The information was gathered and evaluated by the following people: Kimberley Campbell, PharmD, Mary Greene, PharmD, Michael Katz, PharmD, Cindy M. Maggio, PharmD, Teresa C. Nord, PharmD, and Kari Wieland, PharmD.

MEDICATION INDEX

Generic	Trade Names
Acyclovir (PO, IV, and Topical)	Zovirax
Alfa-Interferon	Intron-A, Roferon A
Amikacin	Amikin
Amphotericin B	Fungizone
Atovaquone	Mepron
Azithromycin	Zithromax
Clarithromycin	Biaxin
Clindamycin	Cleocin
Clofazimine	Lamprene
Clotrimazole (PO and Topical)	Mycelex
Dapsone	Dapsone
Didanosine (ddI)	Videx
Diphenoxylate with Atropine	Lomotil
Dronabinol (THC derivative)	Marinol
Erythropoietin	Epogen, Procrit
Ethambutol	Myambutol
Filgrastim	Neupogen
Fluconazole	Diflucan

Folinic Acid	Leucovorin
Foscarnet	Foscavir
Ganciclovir	Cytovene
Isoniazid (INH)	Laniazid, Nydrazid
Itraconazole	Sporanox
Ketoconazole (PO and Topical)	Nizoral
Loperamide	Imodium
Megestrol Acetate	Megace
Methylphenidate	Ritalin
Metronidazole	Flagyl
Morphine Sulfate (MS Contin, MS suppositories)	MS Contin
Nystatin	Mycostatin, Nilstat
Octreotide	Sandostatin
Opium, Tincture of	Tincture of opium
Paramomycin	Humatin
Pentamidine (IV and Inhaled)	Pentam 300, Nebupent
Primaquine	Primaquine
Pyrazinamide	Pryazinamide
Pyrimethamine	Daraprim
Quinolones	Cipro, Noroxin, Floxin
Rifabutin	Mycobutin
Rifampin	Rifadin, Rimactane
Silver Sulfadiazine	Silvadene
Stavudine	Zerit
Streptomycin	Streptomycin
Sulfadiazine	Sulfadiazine
Trimethoprim/Sulfamethoxazole	Bactrim, Septra
Trimetrexate	Neutrexin
Vinblastine	Velban, Velsor
Zalcitabine	Hivid
Zidovudine	Retrovir

VACCINES

Influenza	Fluogen, Fluzone, Flu-imune
Pneumococcus	Pneumovax 23, Pnu-Immune 23

MEDICATIONS

ACYCLOVIR (PO/IV)

Brand Name: Zovirax.

Class: Antimicrobial, antiviral agent.

Indications: Herpes simplex virus, Varicella-zoster virus, Hairy leukoplakia, and Epstein-Barr virus.

Dose: Genital herpes–200 mg PO Q 4 hours 5 times daily x 10 days (primary) or 5 days (recurrent). Herpes Zoster–800 mg PO Q 4 hours 5 times daily. Suppression of chronic HSV–200 mg PO TID or 400 mg PO BID. Severe HSV (including esophageal) 5.0 mg/kg IV Q 8 hours for 7–10 days. Complicated zoster and herpes simplex encephalitis–10 mg/kg IV Q 8 hours for 10 days.

Dose Forms: 200 capsules and 800 mg tablets, 500 and 1000 mg vials for injection, and 200 mg/5 ml suspension.

Side Effects: Arthralgias, diarrhea, headache, nausea/vomiting, and dizziness. Psychosis can be seen at high intravenous doses.

Drug Interactions: In combination with zidovudine, severe drowsiness and lethargy may occur, but an increase in antiretroviral activity has been seen. Probenecid increases the half-life of acyclovir by decreasing its excretion. In combination with alpha-interferon, an increased antiviral activity was seen in vitro. In combination with nephrotoxic drugs, an increased risk of nephrotoxicity exists. High IV doses in combination with other bone-marrow suppressant agents may induce blood dyscrasias (ie, high-dose trimethoprim/sulfamethoxazole).

Important Points: Capsules should be taken with meals at evenly spaced intervals. Decrease intravenous dose in renal dysfunction. Infuse over 1 hour to decrease renal toxicity. May cause phlebitis. Dose should not exceed 500 mg/m^2 Q 8 hours.

Cost: 200 mg capsules $88.40/No.100 or $44.00/10 day treatment; 800 mg tablets $347.32/100, $173.50/10 day treatment. For prophylaxis: 200 mg TID to 400 mg BID monthly cost is $76.64–$106.08

ACYCLOVIR (TOPICAL)

Brand Name: Zovirax.
Class: Antimicrobial, antiviral agent.
Indications: Herpes simplex and genitalia.
Dose: Apply to lesions Q 3 hours 6 times daily for 1 week.
Dose Forms: (5%) 50 mg/gram of drug in 3 and 15 gram tubes.
Side Effects: Pain, burning, and stinging.
Drug Interactions: None.
Important Points: Skin may become hypersensitive with subsequent use. Start therapy as soon as symptoms occur. Oral therapy is considered more effective.
Cost: 3 gram tube is $7.80; 15 gram tube is $18.09.

ALFA-INTERFERON 2A AND 2B

Brand Name: 2b-Intron A, 2a-Roferon A.
Dosage Forms: 2b=3, 18, and 36 million IU vials.
Indications: AIDS's related Kaposi's sarcoma in patients older than 18 years of age. Studies have demonstrated a greater likelihood of response to interferon therapy in patients who are without systemic symptoms, who have limited lymphadenopathy and who have higher CD4 cells.
Dose: Intron A is dosed at 30 mIU/m^2, 3 times weekly subcutaneously or intramuscularly. Continue therapy until there is no further evidence of tumor or infection; adverse reactions require discontinuation. Roferons' induction dose is 36 mIU daily for 10–12 weeks intramuscularly or intravenously. Maintenance dose is 36 mIU 3 times weekly. Dose reductions by half or withholding of individual doses may be required when severe adverse reactions occur. May give as escalating dose schedule at 3, 9, and 18 mIU daily for 3 days followed by an induction period. This has produced equivalent therapeutic benefit and decreased side effects.
Side Effects: Flulike syndrome, fatigue, anorexia, dry mouth, fever, headache, and dyspnea. The incidence of side effects increase in patients receiving larger doses. May see

abnormal white blood cell counts, granulocyte counts, and liver enzyme levels.

Drug Interactions: Not fully evaluated or known. Caution should be exercised when administering interferon in combination with other potentially myelosuppressive agents. Interferon alpha 2a may decrease aminophylline clearance. Zidovudine may increase incidence of neutropenia.

Important Points: Lesion measurements and blood counts should be performed prior to initiation of therapy and should be monitored periodically during treatment or until disease stabilization has occurred. After disease stabilization or response to treatment occurs, treatment should continue until there is no further evidence of tumor or until discontinuation is required because of a severe opportunistic infection or adverse effect. May pretreat with acetaminophen or nonsteroidal anti-inflammatory agents for side effects.

Cost: Intron-A is $9.60/mU, 30 mU SC three times weekly $3456/month; Roferon-A is $9.00/mU; 36 mU SC three times weekly $3888/month.

AMIKACIN

Brand Name: Amikin.

Class: Antimicrobial, aminoglycoside antibiotic.

Indications: *Mycobacterium avium*-intracellulare (MAC) and multidrug resistant *Mycobacterium tuberculosis* (MTB).

Dose: MAC–7.5 mg/kg QD or BID intravenously or intramuscularly for 1 month as part of combination therapy. MTB–7.5 mg/kg BID daily intravenously or intramuscularly 5 days/week for 2 months as part of combination therapy.

Dose Forms: 100 mg/2 ml vial, 500 mg/2 ml syringe, 500 mg/2 ml vial, and 1 gm/4 ml vial.

Side Effects: Nephrotoxicity and ototoxicity.

Drug Interactions: Avoid using with other nephrotoxic drugs such as amphotericin B, vancomycin, loop diuretics, and other aminoglycosides. Avoid using with other ototoxic drugs. May potentiate the effects of neuromuscular blockers.

Important Points: Monitor BUN and creatinine. Dose

according to creatinine clearance. Check levels (peak 20–25 mcg/ml, trough less than 10 mcg/ml and therapeutic range 8–16 mcg/ml) except in QD treatment for MAC. Consider baseline audiometric testing.

Cost: 500 mg/2 ml No.10 vials $637.50; monthly cost is $1912.50.

AMPHOTERICIN B

Brand Name: Fungizone.

Class: Antimicrobial, antifungal agent.

Indications: Disseminated, invasive, and resistant candidiasis, coccidioidomycosis, *Cryptococcus* infection, and histoplasmosis.

Dose: May start with 0.2 mg/kg and increase dose by 0.2 mg/kg/day to about 0.5–1.0 mg/kg/day (1.0 mg test doses are obsolete). After a total dose of 500 mg, the patient may be discharged and continue with 0.5 mg–1 mg/kg 3 times weekly until a total of 1.0 or 2.0 grams has been given or continuation of therapy with fluconazole is appropriate. Continue maintenance dose of 0.5 mg/kg once weekly or change to oral fluconazole. An alternative method for outpatient therapy has been used by Dr. E. Petersen at the University of Arizona. A test dose of 5.0 mg in 50 cc D5W over 1 hour is given in a clinic setting. If tolerated, a dose of 50 mg in 500 cc D5W is given over 2–3 hours in the clinic on the same day. The drug is then continued at this dose 3 times weekly at home until a target cumulative dose is reached (usually 1–2 grams). Appropriate maintenance therapy is required.

Dose Forms: 50 mg vial.

Side Effects: Dose limiting nephrotoxicity, fever, chills, nausea/vomiting, generalized pain especially in the joints and muscles, anorexia, and headache. Thrombocytopenia can also be a side effect.

Drug Interactions: In combination with steroids, hypokalemia can occur. Because of the hypokalemia that may occur, concurrent administration with digoxin is not recommended unless close monitoring occurs. Ticarcillin and carbenicillin exacerbate the hypokalemia. Other nephrotoxic drugs may pose problems.

Important Points: Total cumulative dose should not exceed 4 grams. Monitor BUN, creatinine, and electrolytes. Pre-and postdose sodium loading with 500 cc normal saline may prevent associated nephrotoxocity. Pretreatment with acetaminophen and the addition of 100 units of heparin and 25 mg of hydrocortisone in each bag to prevent phlebitis and fever, respectively, is recommended, although these agents are not necessary. Meperidine may be given for chills and antiemetics for nausea. Beware of normeperidine metabolite accumulation in patients with renal insufficiency who are at risk for seizures. Alternate day therapy may decrease anorexia and phlebitis.

Cost: 50 mg vial $34.89/day 500 mg course $348.90.

ATOVAQUONE (ACUVEL, BW-566C80)

Brand Name: Mepron.
Class: Antimicrobial, antiprotozoal agent.
Indications: *Pneumocystis carinii* pneumonia (PCP).
Dose: 750 mg 3 times a day for 21 days.
Dose Forms: 250 mg tablet.
Side Effects: Rash, fever, headache, nausea, diarrhea, and elevations in liver enzymes.

Drug Interactions: Exercise caution when using with other drugs because there is a potential for interactions resulting from competition for protein binding sites.

Important Points: Atovaquone is second-line therapy for mild-to-moderate PCP in patients intolerant of, or unresponsive to, trimethoprim/sulfamethoxazole. Atovaquone should be administered with food to increase oral absorption and therapeutic efficacy. Currently atovaquone is not indicated for PCP prophylaxis.

Cost: 250 mg No.200 $511.20; 21-day treatment $483.08.

AZITHROMYCIN

Brand Name: Zithromax.
Class: Antimicrobial, macrolide antibiotic.
Indications: In combination with other medications for *Mycobacterium avium*-intracellulare (MAC).
Dose: 500–1000 mg daily for a variable amount of time.
Dose Forms: 250 mg tablets.
Side Effects: Nausea, diarrhea, abdominal pain, and ototoxicity (CNS).
Drug Interactions: Aluminum or magnesium antacids can alter absorption. May enhance prothrombonemic effect of warfarin. Also may increase levels of theophylline, carbamazepine, phenytoin, and triazolam.
Important Points: Patients should take it on an empty stomach. Instruct the patient not to take with aluminum or magnesium containing antacids. Monitor liver enzymes. Do not administer as single agent therapy because of likelihood of drug resistance.
Cost: 250 mg tablets No.30 $234.00 or No.50 $390.00 at 1 gram daily dose $936.00/month.

CLARITHROMYCIN

Brand Name: Biaxin.
Class: Antimicrobial, macrolide antibiotic.
Indications: In combination with other medications for *Mycobacterium avium*-intracellulare (MAC).
Dose: 500–1000 mg Q 12 hours.
Dose Forms: 250 and 500 mg tablets.
Side Effects: Headache, diarrhea, nausea, abnormal taste sensation, and ototoxicity (CNS).
Drug Interactions: Increases blood levels of carbamazepine and theophylline.
Important Points: May be taken without regards to meals. Adjust doses or prolong dosing interval in patients with severe renal impairment.

Cost: 250 or 500 mg tablets No.60 $160.36 at 2 grams daily dose $320.72/month.

CLINDAMYCIN

Brand Name: Cleocin.
Class: Antimicrobial, lincomycin antibiotic.
Indications: *Pneumocystis carinii* pneumonia (PCP) in conjunction with primaquine and toxoplasmosis in conjunction with pyrimethamine.
Dose: 900–1200 mg intravenously Q 8 hours or 450–600 mg orally QID with primaquine for PCP or pyrimethamine for toxoplasmosis.
Dosage Forms: 75 and 150 mg capsules and 300, 600, and 900 mg vials for injection.
Side Effects: Nausea/vomiting, diarrhea, rash, and pseudomembranous colitis (*C difficile,* more common with oral therapy).
Drug Interactions: Kaolin-pectin may reduce absorption from the GI tract. Erythromycin and clindamycin antagonize each other in vitro. May enhance the effects of neuromuscular agents.
Important Points: Patients should inform physician if diarrhea occurs. Each dose should be taken with a full glass of water.
Cost: 150 mg capsules No.100 $103.73; at 300 mg Q 6 hour $248.95/month.

CLOFAZIMINE

Brand Name: Lamprene.
Class: Antimicrobial, leprostatic agent.
Indications: *Mycobacterium avium* complex (MAC).
Dose: 100 mg PO QD.
Dose Forms: 50 and 100 mg capsules.
Side Effects: Reversible discoloration of skin, urine, sweat, and feces, abdominal pain, nausea, increased liver

enzymes, skin dryness, rash, itching, and diarrhea.
Drug Interactions: Dapsone may inhibit the activity of clofazimine.
Important Points: Should be used in combination with other antimycobacterials. Needs to be taken with food. Apply oil to the skin if skin dryness and ichthyosis occur. Monitor liver enzymes. May take months to years for skin discoloration to disappear once therapy is concluded.
Cost: 100 mg capsules No.100 $21.24 at 100 mg daily $6.37/month.

CLOTRIMAZOLE TROCHE

Brand Name: Mycelex Troche.
Class: Antimicrobial, antifungal agent.
Indications: Oropharyngeal candidiasis.
Dose: One troche dissolved in mouth 5 times daily
Dose Forms: 10 mg troche.
Side Effects: Rarely, elevated liver enzymes and nausea/vomiting.
Drug Interactions: None.
Important Points: For best results, the troche must be dissolved slowly in the mouth.
Cost: 10 mg troches No.70 $48.63; $48.63 treatment for 14 days; Prophylaxis at 1 troche TID $62.52/month.

CLOTRIMAZOLE CREAM

Brand Name: Mycelex and Lotrimin.
Class: Antimicrobial, antifungal agent.
Indications: Cutaneous fungal infections.
Dose: Apply BID.
Dose Forms: 1% cream in 12, 15, 30, 45, and 90 gram tubes.
Side Effects: Erythema, stinging, blistering, peeling, and general irritation.
Drug Interactions: None.
Important Points: Patients should apply after cleansing

the area. Clinical improvement with relief of pruritus will occur within a week.

Cost: $9.80/15 gram tube, $16.75/30 gram tube.

DAPSONE (DDS)

Brand Name: Dapsone.
Class: Antimicrobial, leprostatic agent.
Indications: PCP treatment and prophylaxis.
Dose: 100 mg PO 3 QD.
Dose Forms: 25 and 100 mg tablets.
Side Effects: Nausea/vomiting, hemolytic anemia, agranulocytosis, methemoglobinemia, peripheral neuropathy, and phototoxicity.

Drug Interactions: Rifampin increases dapsone clearance. Pyrimethamine and primaquine increases the risk of hematologic toxicity. Probenecid decreases urinary excretion. Zidovudine may increase the bone-marrow toxicity. Didanosine decreases dapsone absorption. The clearance of trimethoprim may be decreased. Phenytoin's half-life will be increased. Patients on warfarin may have an increase in PT. Para-aminobenzoic acid may antagonize dapsone effect.

Important Points: May be used as PCP treatment or prophylaxis in patients with a sulfonamide allergy or hypersensitivity (except in severe cases such as Stevens-Johnsons syndrome). Check Glucose-6-phosphate dehydrogenase (G-6-PD) levels in blacks and people of Eastern Mediterranean descent. Instruct patients to take with food and separate doses of didanosine and dapsone by 2 hours. Requires acidic medium for best absorption. Monitor blood counts. Patients may have increased sensitivity to sunlight.

Cost: 25 mg tablets No.100 $17.20, 100 mg tablets No.60 $17.20; $5.40/month at 100 mg tablet daily.

DIDANOSINE (DDI)

Brand Name: Videx.
Class: Antimicrobial, antiretroviral agent.

Indications: HIV infection.

Dose: > 60 kg: 2 100-mg tabs PO BID. < 60 kg: 1 25-mg tab plus 1 100-mg tab PO BID.

Dose Forms: 25, 50, 100, and 150 mg tablets. 100, 167, 250, and 375 mg single-dose packets.

Side Effects: Dose-limiting peripheral neuropathy, pancreatitis, hepatitis, headache, diarrhea, asymptomatic hyperuricemia, and insomnia.

Drug Interactions: Decreases the absorption of dapsone, ketoconazole, quinolones, and tetracycline. Ganciclovir and intravenous pentamidine may increase the risk of pancreatitis.

Important Points: It is important to note that 2 tablets are required for complete buffering and absorption. Tablets must be chewed or crushed and dissolved in a small amount of water. Following tablets with 8 ounces of water is recommended. Patients should be instructed to take didanosine and dapsone at least 2 hours apart and on an empty stomach. Decrease the dose in patients with renal dysfunction. May need to monitor magnesium in renal dysfunction because each tablet contains 15.7 mEq/tablet. Each tablet has 264.5 mg of sodium

Cost: 25 mg chewable tablets No.60 $21.61, 100 mg chewable tablets No.60 $86.42; 200 mg BID $172.84/month, 125 mg BID $108.03/month.

DIPHENOXYLATE WITH ATROPINE

Brand Name: Lomotil, Lofene, Lomodix, Lonox, Low-Quel, and Lomonate.

Class: Antidiarrheal.

Indications: Diarrhea not a result of *E coli, Salmonella, Shigella,* or *C. difficile.*

Dose: 5.0 mg (2 tabs) orally as needed to control diarrhea (maximum dose is 20.0 mg/day).

Dose Forms: 2.5/0.025 mg diphenoxylate/atropine tablets, same amount in 5 ml of liquid.

Side Effects: Dry skin, flushing, tachycardia, abdominal discomfort, dry mouth, drowsiness, dizziness, toxic megacolon, and urinary retention.

Drug Interactions: Monoamine oxidase inhibitors taken concurrently with diphenoxylate can precipitate a hypertensive crisis. The depressant effects of alcohol, barbiturates, and tranquilizers can be potentiated.

Important Points: If diarrhea is not controlled after 10 days of 20 mg/day, it is unlikely to be controlled by this medication. Loperamide may be more effective. Maintenance doses may be as low as 5.0 mg/day. Patients should avoid alcohol and drink lots of water.

Cost: 2.5 mg tablets No.100 $1.92; at maximum dosing $5.00/month.

DRONABINOL

Brand Name: Marinol.

Class: Antiemetic.

Indications: AIDS wasting syndrome or treatment of nausea/vomiting refractory to conventional antiemetic therapy.

Dose: 2.5 mg PO BID has been effective in AIDS associated wasting syndrome.

Dose Forms: 2.5, 5, and 10 mg capsules.

Side Effects: Profound changes in mental status, dizziness, drowsiness, headache, nausea/vomiting.

Drug Interactions: Do not give with other CNS depressants such as alcohol, sedatives, or hypnotics.

Important Points: Because of the profound effects on the central nervous system, warn patients not to drive, operate complex machinery, or engage in any activity requiring sound judgement and unimpaired coordination. Can persist in tissues and the plasma for days. Can be physically and psychologically addictive. Limit supply. Maximum dose 20 mg/day in divided doses.

Cost: 2.5 mg capsules No.25 $72.22; $173.32/month at minimum dosing.

ERYTHROPOIETIN, EPOETIN ALFA, EPO

Brand Name: Epogen, Procrit.

Dosage Forms: 2,000, 3,000, 4,000, and 10,000 units/ml vials.

Indications: Treatment of anemia related to therapy with AZT in HIV-infected patients. It is used to elevate or maintain the red blood cell level and to decrease the need for transfusions when endogenous erythropoietin level < 500 mU/ml and the dose of AZT is less than 4200 mg/week.

Dose: Initial dose is 100 U/kg as an IV or SQ injection 3 times a week for 8 weeks. If the response is not satisfactory after 8 weeks of therapy, the dose can be increased by 50–200 U/kg 3 times weekly. Evaluate response every 4–8 weeks thereafter and adjust the dose accordingly by 50–100 U/kg 3 times weekly. If patients have not responded satisfactorily to a 300 U/kg dose 3 times weekly, it is unlikely that they will respond to higher doses. When the desired response is attained, titrate the dose to maintain the hematocrit about 30%. If the hematocrit exceeds 40%, discontinue the dose until the hematocrit drops to 36%. When resuming treatment, reduce the dose by 25%, then titrate to maintain desired hematocrit.

Side Effects: Fever, headache, cough, shortness of breath, respiratory congestion, nausea, rash, skin reaction (at injection site). Seizures appear to be related to underlying disease. Hypertension is common in renal failure patients receiving EPO, but does not appear common in AIDS patients.

Drug Interactions: Unknown

Important Points: Prior to beginning therapy, determine the endogenous serum erythropoietin level before transfusing the patient. Evidence suggests that patients receiving AZT with endogenous serum erythropoietin levels > 500 mU/ml are unlikely to respond to therapy. Prior to and during therapy, evaluate the patients' iron stores, include transferrin saturation (should be at least 20%) and serum ferritin (should be at least 100 mg/ml). Monitor hematocrit weekly during the dose adjustment phase of therapy. Patients may need oral iron supplementation during therapy. If the patient is not responding or has a decreased response, the physician may need to check for other sources of anemia, such as folate or vitamin B_{12} deficiencies.

Cost: Epogen^R–vials-2000 U No.10 $240.00, 3000 U No.10 $360.00, 4000 U No.10 $480.00; 10,000 U No.10

$1200.00; 3000 U SC TIW $288/month; 10,000 U SC TIW $1440/month. Procrit^R–vials-2000 U No.6 $144.00, 3000 U No.6 $216.00, 4000 U No.6 $288.00, 10,000 U No.6 $684.00; 3000 U SC TIW $432/month; 4000 U sq TIW $576/month; 10,000 U SC TIW $1365/month.

ETHAMBUTOL

Brand Name: Myambutol.

Class: Antimicrobial, antimycobacterial agent.

Indications: *Mycobacterium avium* complex (MAC) and *Mycobacterium tuberculosis* (MTB).

Dose: 15–25 mg/kg/day PO (not more than 2000 mg daily). 50 mg/kg (maximum 2.5 g twice weekly direct observed therapy (DOT)).

Dose Forms: 100 and 400 mg tablets.

Side Effects: Increased uric acid levels, increased liver enzymes, optic neuritis, peripheral neuritis, headache, dizziness, and nausea/vomiting.

Drug Interactions: Aluminum salts may delay and reduce absorption.

Important Points: Decrease dose with renal dysfunction. Instruct patients to take a single daily dose with food to prevent GI upset. Watch for changes in vision. Monitor periodic renal, hepatic, and hematopoietic systems during long-term therapy.

Cost: 400 mg tablets No.100 $133.86; $99.75/month at 1 gm daily.

FILGRASTIM

Brand Name: Neupogen.

Class: Blood modifier.

Indications: To decrease the incidence of infection associated with febrile neutropenia. To counteract drug-induced neutropenic episodes associated with myelosuppressive agents. Used in idiopathic neutropenia in HIV disease (not FDA-approved for this indication).

Dose: 5 mcg/kg/day SC or IV.

Dosage Forms: 300 mcg/ml, 1 ml and 1.6 ml vials.

Side Effects: Leukocytosis 2%; medullary bone pain 24%, and subclinical and clinical sp splenomegaly seen in 33% and 3%, respectively of patients on chronic therapy. Exacerbation of preexisting skin conditions (psoriasis), alopecia, osteoporosis hematuria/proteinuria and thrombocytopenia (platelets < 50,000/μg) seen less frequently.

Drug Interactions: None listed.

Important Points: For use in HIV-induced idiopathic neutropenia, maintenance of ANC > 1000/μg is targeted (community standard), versus ANC 10,000/μg as seen in oncology patients receiving myelosuppressive agents. Store in refrigerator and discard any vial left at room temperature for > 6 hours. Monitor CBC with differential routinely.

Cost: 300 mcg/ml 1ml vial No.1 $135.00, 1.6 ml $214.00; For maintenance 300 mcg sq QD $4050.00/month.

FLUCONAZOLE

Brand Name: Diflucan.

Class: Antifungal.

Indications: Oropharyngeal, esophageal, and systemic *candidiasis, coccidioidomycosis,* or *cryptococcal* infections.

Dose: Oral Candida–100–200 mg PO QD or QOD. Esophageal Candida–200–400 mg PO QD. Cryptococcus and Cocci suppression–200–400 mg PO QD.

Dosage Forms: 50, 100, and 200 mg tablets and 200 and 400 mg vials for injection.

Side Effects: Nausea/vomiting, diarrhea, abdominal pain, rash, increased liver enzymes, and headache.

Drug Interactions: Rifampin increases metabolism. The metabolism of phenytoin and warfarin are decreased. Increased hypoglycemia with sulfonylureas. Hydrochlorothiazide decreases renal clearance. Cimetidine reduces serum concentrations.

Cyclosporine accumulation may occur.

Important Points: Decrease the dose in renal impairment.

Cost: Maintenance 100 mg PO QD $206.25/month, 200 mg QD $337.50/month.

FOLINIC ACID (LEUCOVORIN)

Brand Name: Leucovorin and Wellcovorin.

Class: Miscellaneous.

Indications: Treatment or prevention of toxicity of folic acid antagonists.

Dose: 5–20 mg/day orally (higher doses may be required).

Dose Forms: 3, 5, and 50 mg per vial for injection, 5 and 25 mg tablets, and oral solution 1 mg/ml.

Side Effects: Allergic sensitization.

Drug Interactions: An increase in seizure frequency may occur with phenytoin. Phenytoin, sulfasalazine, and primidone decrease serum folate levels and produce symptoms of folic acid deficiency.

Important Points: Dose should be increased in patients with bone marrow toxicity. Prophylaxis is not needed with low-dose TMP/SMX in most patients. Daily doses of 5 mg during high-dose TMP/SMX and at all regimens of pyrimethamine and sulfadiazine are recommended.

Cost: 5 mg tablets No.100 $285.00, $85.50/month at 5 mg/day.

FOSCARNET

Brand Name: Foscavir.

Class: Antimicrobial, antiviral.

Indications: Cytomegalovirus and acyclovir-resistant herpes.

Dose: 60 mg/kg Q 8 for induction for 14–21 days.

Maintenance dose may be 90–120 mg/day intravenously. Lower doses are advised for acyclovir-resistant herpes. Dose is adjusted for renal function according to manufacturers recommendations.

Dose Forms: 24 mg/ml in 250 and 500 ml vials.

Side Effects: Nausea, diarrhea, anemia, thrombocytopenia, fever, acute renal failure, seizures, hyper/hypocalcemia, hypokalemia, hypomagnesemia, hyper/hypophosphatemia, and genital ulcers.

Drug Interactions: Drugs that inhibit renal tubular secretion inhibit elimination. The risk of nephrotoxicity increases with amphotericin B, intravenous pentamidine, and aminoglycosides. IV pentamidine increases the risk of hypocalcemia.

Important Points: Give maintenance infusion over 2 hours. Treatment doses should be infused over 1 hour. All doses should be infused via controlled-rate infusion device. Monitor BUN, creatinine, and electrolytes especially ionized calcium. Discontinue at creatinine clearance < 0.4 mg/min/kg. Sodium loading recommended to prevent nephrotoxicity. Normal saline preferred. Electrolyte replacement important. Patients should have eyesight monitored carefully because foscarnet does not cure CMV retinitis. May avoid or treat neutropenia by administering either G-CSF or GM-CSF.

Cost: 250 ml vials $73.28, 500 ml vial $145.93; Maintenance dosing–approximately $2200/month if prepared utilizing each 500 mg vial for > 1 dose (approximately 2 doses/vial for 70 kg patient).

GANCICLOVIR (DHPG)

Brand Name: Cytovene.

Class: Antimicrobial, antiviral agent.

Indications: Cytomegalovirus and acyclovir-resistant herpes.

Dose: Induction: 5.0 mg/kg IV Q 12 hours for 14 to 21 days. Maintenance: 5.0 mg/kg IV seven days/week or 6.0 mg/kg IV 5 days/week.

Dose Forms: 500 mg per vial for injection.

Side Effects: Dose-limiting granulocytopenia and thrombocytopenia, skin rash, phlebitis, fatigue, and nervousness.

Drug Interactions: Neutropenia is seen with zidovudine. Amphotericin B, antineoplastic agents, and flucytosine (5-FC) can increase bone-marrow toxicity. Pancreatitis with didanosine. Imipenem-cilastatin can increase CNS toxicity. Probenecid can decrease the clearance.

Important Points: *Discontinue zidovudine while taking ganciclovir.* Monitor blood counts frequently to monitor for anemia and neutropenia. Manufacturer recommends discontinuing drug in patients with ANC < 500/µg or platelets < 25,000/µg. Decrease dose with renal dysfunction. Infusion should be given over 1 hour. Viral resistance has been reported. Patients should receive adequate hydration during therapy.

Cost: 500 mg vial No.25 $870.00; Maintenance dose–$696.00/month at 5 days/week protocol, $1044/month at daily dosing.

ISONIAZID (INH)

Brand Name: Laniazid and Nydrazid.
Class: Antimycobacterial.
Indications: *Mycobacterium tuberculosis* (MTB).
Dose: 300 mg PO QD; 15 mg/kg (maximum 900 mg) twice weekly DOT.
Dose Forms: 50, 100, and 300 mg tablets, 50 mg/5 ml syrup, and 100 mg/ml (10 ml) vials.
Side Effects: Hepatitis, peripheral neuropathy, skin rash, and nausea/vomiting.
Drug Interactions: Acetaminophen, carbamazepine, and phenytoin have decreased metabolism. Ketoconazole levels may be decreased. Rifampin alters the metabolism. Aluminum salts decrease absorption. Cycloserine increases CNS toxicity. Alcohol increases the risk of hepatitis.
Important Points: Peripheral neuropathy may be treated with pyridoxine (vitamin B6) 50 mg/day. Instruct patients to take this medication on an empty stomach and avoid tyramine

containing foods and alcohol. Monitor liver function tests and ophthalmic exams. Increased sensitivity to isoniazid may occur 3 to 7 weeks after starting treatment, watch for fever, chills, and skin rash.

Cost: 300 mg tablets No.100 $6.34; < $1.00/month.

ITRACONAZOLE

Brand Name: Sporanox.

Class: Antimicrobial, antifungal.

Indications: Treatment of systemic fungal infections including nonmeningeal *Histoplasmosis* and pulmonary and extrapulmonary Blastomycosis for which it is FDA-approved. Demonstrates activity against *Candida, Cryptococcus,* and *Aspergillus.*

Dose: 200 mg PO QD - BID **with meals.** In severe infections, a loading dose of 200 mg PO TID may be administered for 3 days. Doses exceeding 200 mg should be divided into 2 daily doses.

Dosage Forms: 100 mg capsules.

Side Effects: Itraconazole is structurally similar to other triazole derivatives such as fluconazole and terconazole, with similar side effect profiles. Hepatitis has been reported in 4 patients, 3 with an idiosyncratic reaction. Nausea, vomiting, and diarrhea have also been reported. Edema, rash, headache, hypokalemia, and hypertension have been reported. Less frequent side effects include adrenal suppression and gynecomastia.

Drug Interactions: Significant increases in cyclosporine serum concentrations warranting a decrease in cyclosporine dose by 50%. Increases in digoxin and oral sulfonylyrea levels may also occur. Life-threatening ventricular arrhythmias may occur with terfenadine contraindicating concurrent use. Decreased plasma itraconazole levels have been reported with H_2-antagonsits, isoniazid, rifampin, and phenytoin. Phenytoin levels may also be decreased. It is recommended to avoid use of rifampin and itraconazole, as this interaction is felt to significantly impair antifungal efficacy and may result in life-threatening outcomes especially in immunocompromised patients. Increased anticoagulant effects of warfarin may occur.

Important Points: Monitor liver function tests. Warn patients to report GI distress and hepatitis to their physician. Use with caution in patients with history of liver disease. Doses of itraconazole may need to be adjusted, although exact guidelines do not exist.

Cost: 100 mg capsules $147.60/No.30. $295.20/month of 200 mg daily.

KETOCONAZOLE

Brand Name: Nizoral.
Class: Antimicrobial, antifungal agent.
Indications. *Candidiasis*.
Dose: Oral candidiasis–Treatment 200 mg PO QD; MWF for prophylaxis. Esophageal candidiasis–400 mg PO QD for 14 days.
Dose Forms: 200 mg tablets and 100 mg/5 ml suspension.
Side Effects: Hepatotoxicity, nausea/vomiting, diarrhea, abdominal pain, headache, gynecomastia, and adrenal suppression.
Drug Interactions: Antacids, H_2 blockers, anticholinergics, and didanosine decreases ketoconazole bioavailability. Terfenadine can cause life-threatening arrhythmias (contraindicated). Rifampin can increase the metabolism and decrease absorption up to 80%. Isoniazid can also increase the metabolism. May have increased levels of theophylline and anticoagulants. Cyclosporine levels may be increased.
Important Points: Patient should not take antacids within 2 hours of ketoconazole because an acid pH is required for absorption. Instruct patients take with food. Patients who fail ketoconazole may be achlorhydric or have decreased gastric acid secretion. Recommend taking with cola-type soda to decrease gastric pH. Resistant infections may respond to fluconazole. Not recommended for treatment of systemic non-Candidal fungal infections in immunosuppressed patients. **Note:** Recommend taking dose in AM to allow cirdacian testosterone recovery to occur in males in the PM.

Cost: 200 mg tablets No.100 $232.27; 200 mg QD $69.68/month.

KETOCONAZOLE 2% CREAM

Brand Name: Nizoral.
Class: Antimicrobial, topical antifungal.
Indications: Cutaneous fungal infections.
Dose: Apply to affected areas BID or QD.
Dose Forms: 15, 30, and 60 g tube.
Side Effects: Itching, burning, and skin irritation.
Drug Interactions: None.
Important Points: Treatment should continue for 2 weeks after resolution of symptoms.
Cost: 15 g tube $11.59, 30 g tube $19.49; average $19.49–$38.98/month.

LOPERAMIDE

Brand Name: Imodium and Imodium-AD.
Class: Antidiarrheal.
Indications: Diarrhea not associated with *E coli, Salmonella, Shigella,* or *C difficile.*
Dose: Start with 4.0 mg followed by 2.0 mg after each loose stool until controlled. Average daily dose is 4.0–8.0 mg PO. Do not exceed 16 mg/day. Chronic diarrhea may need as much as 2.0–4.0 mg every 6 hours.
Dose Forms: 2 mg tablets or capsules and 1 mg/5 ml liquid.
Side Effects: Abdominal pain or distention, dry mouth, and CNS depression (including drowsiness or dizziness).
Drug Interactions: None.
Important Points: In chronic diarrhea, if no improvement after 16 mg/day for 10 days, then this medication probably will not be effective. If a dose is forgotten, patients may take the medication as soon as they remember and space consecutive doses evenly or skip the dose entirely if diarrhea is not currently a problem.

Cost: 2 mg capsules No.100 $50.57; maximum dosing $121.37/month.

MEGESTROL ACETATE

Brand Name:. Megace

Class: Progesterone derivative, appetite stimulant.

Indications: Appetite stimulant for AIDS patients with severe wasting.

Dose: 80–200 mg PO QID tablets or 800 mg/day suspension (FDA-approved dose and dosage form).

Dose Forms: 20 and 40 mg tablets; 40 mg/ml suspension in 8 oz bottle.

Side Effects: Back or abdominal pain, headache, nausea/vomiting, breast tenderness, hyperpnea, and women may have abnormal vaginal bleeding. Hyperglycemia may also be seen. Women of childbearing age should be advised against becoming pregnant while taking this drug.

Drug Interactions: Not investigated.

Important Points: May be taken with food. At least 1–2 months of continuous therapy may be necessary until full effects of the drug are apparent. It is best to take doses around the clock. New information on suspension recommends 800 mg as a daily dose for 30 days, then 400 mg daily thereafter. Manufacturer recommend 4-month trial. Currently, manufacturer supplying free drug to patients who qualify (1-800-321-1335).

Cost: Using 20 mg tablets-80 mg QID $155.40, 8 oz suspension $61.85, initial 800 mg/day $154.63 then maintenance $77.32/month.

METHYLPHENIDATE

Brand Name: Ritalin and Ritalin-SR.

Class: Antidepressant and CNS stimulant.

Indications: Depression and severe fatigue. May be useful in mild HIV dementia.

Dose: 5.0–20 mg orally BID daily, with the last dose before 6 PM to avoid insomnia.

Dose Forms: 5, 10, and 20 mg tablets.

Side Effects: Insomnia, nervousness, tachycardia, hypertension, anemia, and leukopenia; hallucinations and delirium from overdosage; may worsen underlying psychosis.

Drug Interactions: Other CNS stimulants.

Important Points: Patients should take at least 30–45 minutes prior to meals and before 6 PM. Monitor blood pressure and CBC. Do not crush or chew controlled release tablets. Do not double doses.

Cost: 5 mg tablets No.100 $17.63, 10 mg tablets No.100 $24.75, 20 mg tablets No.100 $37.50; 5 mg BID $10.20/month, 20 mg BID $22.50.

METRONIDAZOLE

Brand Name: Flagyl, Protostat.

Class: Antimicrobial, amebicide.

Indications: Anaerobic infections (ie, *C difficile,* giardiasis, trichomoniasis, *Gardnerella vaginalis.*

Dose: 500 mg PO BID for 7 days for trichomoniaisis or bacterial vaginosis.

Dosage Forms: 250 mg and 500 mg tablets, 500 mg lyophilized vials and 500 mg in 100 ml ready-to-use vials and containers.

Side Effects: CNS, nausea, vomiting, anorexia, metallic taste, some blood dyscrasias, dark urine, flattening of T-wave on ECG, and hypersensitivity.

Drug Interactions: Alcohol will produce an Antabuse-like reaction. Barbiturates can decrease metronidazole therapeutic efficacy and lead to increased anticoagulant effects of warfarin. Decreased clearance of phenytoin with increased elimination half-life. Increased lithium levels and toxicity demonstrated in patients on high-dose lithium.

Important Points: For trichomoniasis, restrict to second and third trimester if possible, for patients in whom local palliative treatment is ineffective. Nursing mothers can resume breast-feeding 24–48 hours after discontinuation of the drug. Breast milk produced during therapy should be expressed and discarded. Use with caution in patients with hepatic impairment. Treatment of sexual partners indicated, especially in symptomatic infection.

Cost: 250 mg tablets No.100 $121.02; 500 mg BID for 7 days $33.89.

MORPHINE SULFATE CONTINUOUS RELEASE

Brand Name: MS Contin, Oramorph SR.

Class: Narcotic analgesic.

Indications: Relief of moderate to severe acute and chronic pain.

Dose: Depends upon required stabilized daily dose of immediate-release formulation divided BID to TID. In patients receiving < 60 mg total daily dose of immediate-release morphine sulfate, it is recommended to use the 15 mg sustained-release tablets. For patients receiving 60–120 mg total daily dose of immediate-release morphine sulfate, it is recommended to use the 30 mg sustained-release tablets. For patients receiving > 120 mg total daily dose of immediate-release morphine sulfate, it is recommended to use the 100 mg dose of sustained-release tablets in combination with the other doses available.

Dosage Forms: MS Contin–tablets 15, 30, 60, and 100 mg Oramorph SR–tablets 30, 60, and 100 mg.

Side Effects: CNS including respiratory and cough suppression, nausea and vomiting, sedation, depression, and mental clouding. Decreased GI motility and biliary spasm (with elevated amylase and lipase concentrations). Orthostatic hypotension and histamine-associated flushing, pruritus, red eyes, and sweating. Miosis can develop in chronic users. Some patients develop insomnia. Morphine sulfate has a high potential for physical addiction.

Drug Interactions: Morphine can potentiate CNS depressant effects of general anesthetics, tranquilizers, other opiate agonists, sedatives, hypnotics, and alcohol. Other CNS drugs including tricyclic antidepressants and MAO inhibitors should be used cautiously and in reduced doses. Phenothiazines may antagonize opiate agonists like morphine.

Important Points: Patients should be stabilized on

immediate-release narcotic analgesics prior to conversion to sustained-release preparation. Addition of stool softener and periodic laxative should be considered as adjunctive therapy to avoid severe constipation or fecal impaction. Do not crush or chew sustained-release preparation because rapid release of morphine may result in a toxic dose. Beware of abrupt discontinuation of opiates, which may cause physical withdrawal.

Cost: MS Contin Tablets: 15 mg No.100 $69.74; 30 mg No.100 $132.52; 60 mg No.100 $258.60; 30 mg BID $79.20/month; 60 mg Q 8 hour $232.74/month.

NYSTATIN

Brand Name: Mycostatin, Nilstat, O-V Statin.

Class: Antimicrobial, topical antifungal agent.

Indications: *Candida* infections, ie, vaginal thrush, intestinal, cutaneous or mucocutaneous infections.

Dose: Vaginal–Insert 1 tablet vaginally at bedtime for 14 days; Topically–Apply to affected area 2–3 times daily; Oral Suspension–400,000–600,000 U swish and swallow 4 times daily for thrush, 1 tablet PO TID for GI infection.

Dosage Forms: Vaginal and Oral Tablets–100,000 U, 500,000 U; Cream, Ointment, and Powder–100,000 U/gram; Oral Suspension–100,000 U/ml.

Side Effects: Hypersensitivity, virtually nontoxic; large oral doses are associated with nausea, vomiting, and elevated liver enzymes.

Drug Interactions: None.

Important Points: For intestinal infection continue therapy for 48 hours after signs and symptoms have completely resolved. For HIV-infected women with recurrent or severe vaginal thrush a minimum of 7 days of treatment is recommended. Additionally, chronic suppressive therapy may be likely in this population with recurrent infections or those receiving antibiotics. **Note:** Vaginal tablets may be used orally like troches.

Cost: Vaginal Tablets 100,000 U (with applicator) No.15 $4.00 and No.30 $6.40/month; Oral Suspension 60 cc $4.60 (generic), 6 cc QID $55.20/month.

OCTREOTIDE

Brand Name: Sandostatin.
Class: Antidiarrheal.
Indications: Refractory secretory diarrhea.
Dose: 50–100 mcg subcutaneously QD, BID or TID.
Dose Forms: 50, 100, and 500 mcg ampules for injection.
Side Effects: Pain or burning at the injection site, abdominal cramping and pain, diarrhea or loose stools, steatorrhea, nausea/vomiting, and postprandial hyperglycemia.
Drug Interactions: Decreased cyclosporine levels. Potentially, an alteration in response to thyroid supplementation and diabetes therapy.
Important Points: None.
Cost: 100 μg/ml No.20 $148.32; 100–500 μg SQ TID $667.44/month to $2002.32/month.

OPIUM, TINCTURE OF

Brand Name: None.
Class: Antidiarrheal, analgesic.
Indications: Diarrhea refractory to other agents.
Dose: 0.6 ml PO QID.
Dose Forms: 10% opium in 19% alcohol as 120 ml or one pint.
Side Effects: Constipation, drowsiness, hypotension, nausea/vomiting, sweating, and dizziness.
Drug Interactions: Anticholinergics may add to the effects of tincture of opium. CNS depressants can have an increased effect.
Important Points: Tolerance to antidiarrheal effects may develop with repeated use. If using chronically, decrease dose slowly to limit withdrawal symptoms. Patient must avoid alcohol. May cause drowsiness. Ensure adequate treatment of infectious diarrhea.
Cost: 4 oz dropper bottle $42.10; $25.20/month.

PARAMOMYCIN

Brand Name: Humatin.
Class: Antimicrobial, amebicide (aminoglycoside).
Indication: Acute and chronic intestinal amebiasis, recalcitrant cryptosporidial diarrhea.
Dose: Cryptosporidiosis–studies have used 500 mg BID to 500–750 mg TID to QID; up to 35 mg/kg/day in 3 divided doses.
Dosage Forms: 250 mg capsules.
Side Effects: Doses > 3 grams associated with nausea, diarrhea, and abdominal cramps.
Drug Interactions: Although GI absorption is poor, increased risks of ototoxicity and nephrotoxicity in combination with other ototoxic (other aminoglycoside antibiotics, furosemide) and nephrotoxic (aminoglycosides, amphotericin B, vancomycin, etc) agents exists.
Important Points: Increased absorption possible through ulcerative bowel. Counsel patients to notify physician of dizziness, tinnitus, or hearing impairment. Treatment not highly effective for this infection.
Cost: 250 mg capsules No.16 $27.61; 500 mg BID $207.08/month, 750 mg QID $621.23/month.

PENTAMIDINE (IV)

Brand Name: Pentam 300.
Class: Antimicrobial, antiprotozoal agent.
Indications: *Pneumocystis carinii* infection.
Dose: 4.0 mg/kg IV QD.
Dose Forms: 300 mg vials.
Side Effects: Nephrotoxicity, hypotension, hyper/hypoglycemia, hyperkalemia, leukopenia, thrombocytopenia, increased liver enzymes, neuralgias, dizziness, nausea/vomiting, insulin-requiring diabetes, pancreatitis, and metallic taste.
Drug Interactions: Nephrotoxic drugs (ie, amphotericin B, aminoglycosides, and vancomycin) and foscarnet can

increase the risk of nephrotoxicity. Foscarnet can also cause severe hypocalcemia.

Important Points: Educate patient about hypoglycemia that can occur approximately 5–7 days into therapy (earlier or later is also possible). Administer intravenously over at least 1 hour to decrease hypotension. Monitor liver enzymes and potassium. Hydrate regularly. Administering this drug during morning hours is recommended to decrease effects on glucose metabolism and associated side effects that may go unnoticed during the night. Morning finger sticks before dose is also advised.

Cost: 300 mg vial No.1 $85.00; 21-day course $1785.00.

PENTAMIDINE (INHALED)

Brand Name: Nebupent.

Class: Antimicrobial, antiprotozoal agent.

Indications: *Pneumocystis carinii* pneumonia prophylaxis.

Dose: 300 mg Q 4 weeks via Respirgard II nebulizer, or 60 mg Q 2 weeks by Fisoneb ultrasonic nebulizer (after a loading dose).

Dose Forms: 300 mg aerosol.

Side Effects: Cough, bronchospasm, laryngitis, nausea/vomiting, gingivitis, increased liver enzymes, tremors, confusion, and anxiety. Reports of hypo/hyperglycemia, cardiovascular complications, and conjunctivitis.

Drug Interactions: None.

Important Points: Patients should change position during treatments to allow more complete distribution throughout the lungs. Extrapulmonary *Pneumocystosis* is not prevented by inhalation treatment. Reports of pneumocystis of upper lobes and pneumothorax have been reported in patients on aerosol prophylaxis. Patients should be instructed to wait 5–10 minutes between the use of a bronchodilator and pentamidine.

Cost: 1 vial 300 mg $98.75/month.

PRIMAQUINE

Brand Name: None.
Class: Antimicrobial, antiprotozoal agent.
Indications: *Pneumocystis carinii* pneumonia in conjunction with Clindamycin.
Dose: 15–30 mg/daily of the base.
Dose Forms: 26.3 mg tablets equivalent to 15 mg of base.
Side Effects: Nausea/vomiting, hemolytic anemia in patients with Glucose-6-phosphate dehydrogenase (G-6-PD) deficiency, methemoglobinemia, and bone-marrow suppression.
Drug Interactions: Quinacrine can potentiate the toxicity of antimalarials structurally related to primaquine. Medications causing bone marrow depression can enhance this effect.
Important Points: Patient may take with food if abdominal distress occurs. Black patients and patients of Eastern Mediterranean descent should have their G-6-PD levels checked.
Cost: 26.3 mg tablets No.100 $98.75; 1 tablet daily $29.63/month.

PYRAZINAMIDE

Brand Name: None.
Class: Antimicrobial, antimycobacterial agent.
Indications: *Mycobacterium tuberculosis* (MTB).
Dose: 15–30 mg/kg/day in 1–4 divided doses not to exceed 3.0 grams/day (CDC recommends maximum dose of 2 grams as combination therapy); 50–70 mg/kg (maximum 2 g) twice weekly DOT.
Dose Forms: 500 mg tablets.
Side Effects: Nausea/vomiting, hepatotoxicity, increased uric acid, and arthralgias.
Drug Interactions: Allopurinol, colchicine, probenecid, and ethionamide.

Important Points: Give in combination with other antimycobacterials. Monitor liver enzymes. Patients should notify physician of fever, loss of appetite, malaise, nausea/vomiting, darkened urine, yellowish discoloration of the skin and eyes, or symptoms of gouty arthritis. Recommended not to be used in renal insufficiency (Creatinine clearance < 50 ml/min).

Cost: 500 mg tablets No.100 $92.97; 1500 mg daily $83.67/month.

PYRIMETHAMINE

Brand Name: Daraprim.

Class: Antimicrobial, antiprotozoal agent.

Indications: Treatment of toxoplasmosis in conjunction with sulfadiazine.

Dose: 75–100 mg/daily PO for 6 weeks then decrease to 25–50 mg/daily 3–7 times per week as maintenance.

Dose Forms: 25 mg tablets.

Side Effects: Megaloblastic anemia, thrombocytopenia, leukopenia, anorexia, vomiting, ataxia, tremors, increased liver enzymes, hypersensitivity reaction (urticaria, pruritis, and Stevens-Johnson syndrome).

Drug Interactions: Folic acid antagonists (ie, methotrexate, sulfonamides, trimethoprim-sulfamethoxazole) can cause anemia. AZT can possibly cause an increase in bone marrow suppression. AZT may decrease intracellular pyrimethamine concentrations.

Important Points: Patients should take with food. Monitor blood counts frequently. Patients should discontinue medication if rash develops, and call the physician. Patients should receive folinic acid when pyrimethamine is being administered. Monotherapy for secondary prophylaxis of toxoplasma encephalitis not recommended.

Cost: 25 mg tablets No.100 $34.75; 50 mg daily $20.85.

QUINOLONES

Brand Name: Ciprofloxacin (Cipro), Enoxacin (Penetrex), Lomefloxacin (Maxaquin), Norfloxacin (Noroxin), and Ofloxacin (Floxin).

Class: Antimicrobial, antimycobacterial and antibacterial.

Indications: *Mycobacterium avium*-intracellulare (MAC), *Shigella,* and a variety of bacterial infections.

Doses: Ciprofloxacin: 250–750 mg PO BID (MAC use 750 mg BID); Enoxacin: 200–400 mg PO BID (*N gonorrhoeae* and UTI); Lomefloxacin: 400 mg PO QD (complicated UTI, cystitis, and acute bacterial exacerbation of chronic bronchitis); Norfloxacin: 400 mg PO BID (UTI) and 800 mg PO QD (uncomplicated gonorrhea); Ofloxacin: 200–400 mg PO BID (MAC use 400 mg BID).

Dose Forms: Ciprofloxacin: 250, 500, and 750 mg tablets and 200 and 400 mg injections; Enoxacin: 200 and 400 mg tablets; Lomefloxacin: 400 mg tablets; Norfloxacin: 400 mg tablets; Ofloxacin: 200, 300, and 400 mg tablets and 400 mg and 800 mg vials (4 mg/ml).

Side Effects: Nausea, vomiting, diarrhea, dizziness, and photosensitivity.

Drug Interactions: Antacids, zinc salts, and iron salts interfere with absorption. Probenecid increases the clearance. The clearance of theophylline and caffeine is reduced. Sucralfate can reduce serum Cipro levels significantly.

Important Points: Decrease dose with renal dysfunction. Patients should take with full glass of water and on an empty stomach. This medication must not be taken with antacids or vitamins. Food may decrease absorption of norfloxacin and extent of absorption of lomefloxacin. Patients need to avoid dairy products with ciprofloxacin because of decreased absorption. Precautionary use is necessary in prepubescent children owing to interference with cartilage and long bone growth.

Cost: Ciprofloxacin: 250 mg tablets No.100 $252.54, 500 mg tablets No.100 $292.25, 750 mg tablets No.50 $253.45; 750 mg BID $304.14/month; Enoxacin: 200 mg or 400 mg tablets No.50 $130.00; Lomefloxacin: 400 mg tablets No.20

$113.18; Norfloxacin: 400 mg tablets No.100 $234.21; Ofloxacin: 200 mg tablets No.50 $134.05, 300 mg tablets No.50 $159.60, 400 mg tablets No.50 $168.05.

RIFABUTIN

Brand Name: Mycobutin.
Class: Antimicrobial, antimycobacterial agent.
Indications: Prevention of *Mycobacterium avium* complex (MAC) (FDA approval); Treatment of MAC and *Mycobacterium tuberculosis* (MTB).
Dose: 150–300 mg/day.
Dose Forms: 150 mg capsules.
Side Effects: Rash, gastrointestinal symptoms, uveitis, muscle and joint aches, and discolored urine, sweat, and saliva; additionally, thrombocytopenia, anemia, and hepatotoxicity (although less frequently).
Drug Interactions: Rifampin may increase risk for drug toxicity when given with rifabutin. Rifabutin may increase clearance of cyclosporine. Concurrent antimycobacterial therapy, has the potential to antagonize, or negate, the BCG vaccine-mediated effect of BCG live or BCG vaccine.
Important Points: Adjust dose in suspected bone marrow or hepatotoxicity. Use in combination with other medications for above mentioned indications. May cause discoloration of urine. Monitor cyclosporine blood levels because levels may be decreased. Because of increased risk for drug toxicity rifampin should not be administered with rifabutin. Decreases zidovudine levels but no dose adjustment recommended. Decreases oral contraceptives effectiveness. Should be used in combination with other antimycobacterial agents for treatment of MAC or MTB to prevent resistance.
Cost: 150 mg capsules No.100 $327.00; 300 mg QD $196.20.

RIFAMPIN

Brand Name: Rifadin and Rimactane.
Class: Antimycobacterial.

Indications: *Mycobacterium avium*-intracellulare complex (MAC) and *Mycobacterium tuberculosis* (MTB).

Dose: 10 mg/kg/day PO (maximum 600 mg/day) QD or divided BID; 10 mg/kg (maximum 600 mg) twice weekly DOT.

Dose Forms: 150 and 300 mg capsules, 600 mg injectable.

Side Effects: Flulike symptoms (fever, chills, bone and muscle pain, headache, nausea/vomiting), thrombocytopenia, anemia, acute interstitial nephritis, and liver dysfunction.

Drug Interactions: Rifampin is an enzyme inducer that will decrease effects of acetaminophen, oral contraceptives, dapsone, fluconazole, ketoconazole, steroids, methadone, benzodiazepines, digoxin, coumadin, sulfones, quinidine, theophylline, ketoconazole, trimethoprim, enalapril, and verapamil. A significant interaction with itraconazole has been documented resulting in decreased itraconazole efficacy. Combination may lead to decreased efficacy of itraconazole. Isoniazid and alcohol in conjuction increases the risk of hepatotoxicity.

Important Points: Use in combination with other medications for above mentioned indications. Medication should be taken on an empty stomach with a full glass of water. May cause discoloration of urine, tears, stool, sweat, saliva, and sputum. May stain soft contact lenses. Patients taking methadone may need doses increased by 10 mg every 1–2 days starting the day rifampin is added. Some patients may require a 50% dose increase.

Cost: 150 mg capsules No.30 $42.20, 300 mg capsules No.100 $204.06; 2 × 300 mg $122.44/month.

SILVER SULFADIAZINE

Brand Name: Silvadene and Flint SSD.

Class: Antibiotic, antifungal, and possibly antiviral.

Indications: Dermal wounds infected by *Staphylococcus, Streptococcus,* or *Candida.* Severe herpetic lesions (especially perirectal).

Dose: Apply to affected area BID or QD.

Dose Forms: 20, 50, 400, and 1000 gram tubes at 10 mg/gram of drug.

Side Effects: Photosensitivity and hypersensitivity.
Drug Interactions: None.
Important Points: Caution must be used when administering this drug to patients with allergies to sulfonamides, sulfonylureas, furosemide, thiazide diuretics, and parabens. May discolor skin. Patients should inform physician if any hyperventilation indicating hypersensitivity occurs.
Cost: 50 gram $5.33.

STAVUDINE (D4T)

Brand Name: Zerit.
Class: Antiretroviral.
Indications: Failure of or intolerance to other antiretrovirals.
Dose: < 60 kg: 30 mg BID; > 60 kg: 40 mg BID.
Dose Forms: 15, 20, 30, 40 mg capsules.
Side Effects: Peripheral neuropathy most common. Abnormal liver function tests, granulocytopenia, headache, myopathy, pancreatitis, and hyperamylanemia have been observed in patients receiving stavudine.
Drug Interactions: Not established; possible zidovudine.
Important Points: Adjust dose in renal impairment or if peripheral neuropathy develops.
Cost: Not established.

STREPTOMYCIN

Brand Name: None.
Class: Antimicrobial, antimycobacterial agent.
Indications: *Mycobacterium tuberculosis* (MTB).
Dose: 15 mg/kg/day; 25–30 mg/kg (maximum 1 gram or maximum 750 mg > 60-year-olds) twice weekly DOT.
Dose Forms: 1.0 and 5.0 gram vials at 400 mg/ml.
Side Effects: Nephrotoxicity and ototoxicity.
Drug Interactions: Nephrotoxic or ototoxic medications

may potentiate the toxic effects.

Important Points: Adjust dose in renal impairment. Use in combination with other antimycobacterials. Give as deep intramuscular injection only. Available through Pfizer Streptomycin Program for patients with MDR-TB where sensitivities demonstrate drug indication, or in patients unable to tolerate other available first-line antimycobacterial agents.

Cost: 1 g No.25 $17.25; 1 g IM QD $20.70/month. Available through Pfizer only (see Appendix).

SULFADIAZINE

Brand Name: None.
Class: Antimicrobial, antibiotic agent.
Indications: *Toxoplasmosis* with pyrimethamine.
Dose: 2.0–4.0 grams/day PO divided QID.
Dose Forms: 500 mg tablets.
Side Effects: Nausea, anorexia, diarrhea, headache, peripheral neuropathy, impaired folic acid absorption, leukopenia, thrombocytopenia, methemoglobinemia, erythema multiforme, crystalluria, and photosensitivity.

Drug Interactions: Increases half-life of sulfonylureas, and hypoglycemia has occurred. Methotrexate or trimetrexate-induced bone marrow suppression may be enhanced. The anticoagulation activity of warfarin may be enhanced leading to hemorrhage. Other interactions may be seen with thiazide diuretics, salicylates, probenecid, and phenytoin.

Important Points: This drug should be taken on an empty stomach with a full glass of water. Currently, it is only available through the CDC at (404) 488-4928. Recommend addition of daily leucovorin.

Cost: No cost from CDC at this time.

TRIMETHOPRIM/SULFAMETHOXAZOLE

Brand Name: Bactrim, Bactrim DS, Septra, and various others.
Class: Antimicrobial.

Indications: *Pneumocystis carinii* pneumonia prophylaxis and treatment and antibacterial (UTI or dysentery).

Dose: Prophylaxis–1 double strength (DS) tablet QD or 3 times weekly (MWF); Acute PCP treatment–15–20 mg/kg trimethoprim component divided Q 6 hours PO or IV. Must complete 21 days of therapy.

Dose Forms: Single strength tablet 80 mg TMP and 400 mg SMX. Double strength tablet 160 mg TMP and 800 mg SMX. Oral suspension 40 mg TMP and 200 mg SMX per 5 ml, IV is the same dose as PO.

Side Effects: Rash, itching, photosensitivity, leukopenia, thrombocytopenia, fever, nausea/vomiting, and Stevens-Johnson syndrome, tremors nephrotoxicity, and hyperkalemia associated with trimethoprim.

Drug Interactions: An increase in the hypoglycemic effect may be seen with the sulfonylureas. A decrease in phenytoin's hepatic clearance and an increase in its half-life can be seen. The prothrombin time (PT) may be prolonged in patients taking warfarin. An increase in thrombocytopenia with purpura has been seen in the elderly taking thiazide diuretics. Increases in free methotrexate concentrations can be seen as a result of protein binding displacement, therefore increasing the risk for bone marrow suppression. Other effects can be seen with NSAIDs, probenecid, and salicylates.

Important Points: Patients need to avoid sunlight and take orally with a full glass of water. They may take diphenhydramine for itching and rash. Decrease the dose in renal impairment. Therapeutic peaks of SMX levels should be 75–125 mcg/ml 1 hour after an intravenous and 2 hours after an oral dose. Monitor liver enzymes. Routine administration of folinic acid is not necessary. Five mg of leucovorin daily during treatment of PCP is recommended. Monitor for hyponatremia associated with administration of D5W diluent in IV preparation; may be mixed in normal saline despite decreased stability.

TRIMETREXATE GLUCURONATE

Brand Name: Neutrexin.
Class: Antimicrobial, antiprotozoal agent.
Indications: Treatment of moderate to severe *Pneu-*

mocytis carinii pneumonia in patients intolerant to other first-line agents.

Dose: 45 mg/m^2 IV QD over 60–90 minutes Must be administered concomitantly with leucovorin 20 mg/m^2 IV or PO Q 6 hours. *See package insert for dosage adjustments based upon hematologic toxicity grading system.*

Dosage Forms: 25 mg vials for IV use.

Side Effects: Neutropenia and thrombocytopenia occurs, however, fever, rash, elevated liver enzymes, nephrotoxicity and electrolyte abnormalities have been reported. Nausea and vomiting reported but significantly less than comparative trials with trimethoprim/sulfamethoxazole. Manufacturer states, however, that patients receiving trimetrexate IV may experience severe hematologic, hepatic, renal, and GI toxicities.

Drug Interactions: Bone marrow suppressants, folate antagonists and nephrotoxic agents. Interactions with drugs metabolized by the cytochrome P450 enzyme system including erythromycin, rifampin, rifabutin, ketoconazole and fluconazole may result in altered serum trimetrexate concentrations. Competition for drug clearance and metabolism may also result from concommitant use with cimetidine or acetaminophen.

Important Points: Must be taken with high doses of leucovorin to prevent toxicity to blood cells. Leucovorin should continue 72 hours after last dose of drug. Not first-line therapy. Prophylaxis doses not established. *Pregnancy category D.*

Cost: 21-day treatment course is approximately $2600.

VINBLASTINE (INTRALESIONAL)

Brand Name: Velban, Velsor, Alkaban-AQ.

Class: Antineoplastic.

Dosage Forms: 10 mg/vial of powder for injection and 10 mg/10 ml vials.

Indications: Intralesional treatment of Kaposi's sarcoma.

Dose: 0.1 mg injections into the center of the lesion, not to exceed 2 lesions per treatment (reduce systemic toxicity).

Side Effects: Mucositis may occur with oral lesions. Bone marrow suppression occurs.

Drug Interactions: None.

Important Points: Usually use diluted vinblastine at 0.2 mg/cc, not to exceed 0.5 cc per lesion. Therapy can be repeated every 2 weeks. Inform patients of lesional necrosis.

Cost: 1 mg No.1 $14.50, 5 mg No.1 $32.25, Pdi IV 10 mg No.10 $212.50.

ZALCITABINE (DDC)

Brand Name: HIVID.
Class: Antimicrobial, antiretroviral.
Indications: HIV infection.
Dose: 0.375 mg or 0.750 mg TID.
Dose Forms: 0.375 and 0.75 mg tablets.
Side Effects: Dose related peripheral neuropathy, also pancreatitis, rash, mouth sores, fever, and malaise. These effects should subside after a few months of therapy.

Drug Interactions: Other drugs that cause peripheral neuropathy, ie, ddI and dapsone.

Important Points: Zalcitabine should be discontinued in patients exhibiting moderate discomfort from numbness, tingling, burning, or pain of the extremities with progression. If symptoms resolve to mild intensity, rechallenge with half-dosage may be permitted. Dose should be decreased in patients with impaired renal function.

Cost: 0.375 mg tablets No.100 $170.40, 0.750 mg tablets No.100 $213.60; $153.00–$192.24/month.

ZIDOVUDINE (ZDV)

Brand Name: Retrovir.
Class: Antimicrobial, antiretroviral.
Indications: HIV infection. HIV-related thrombocytopenia and AIDS related dementia may respond to zidovudine.
Dose: 100 mg Q 4 hours 5 times daily or 200 mg TID.
Dose Forms: 100 mg capsules, 50 mg/5 ml syrup, and 10 mg/ml in 20 ml vial for injection.
Side Effects: Granulocytopenia and anemia are dose-

limiting toxicities, headache, nausea/vomiting, fatigue, and myopathy.

Drug Interactions: Ganciclovir has additive hematologic toxicity. TMP/SMX, sulfadiazine, pyrimethamine, amphotericin-B, dapsone, aspirin, and alfa-interferon may cause increased bone marrow or hematologic toxicity. Acyclovir, alfa-interferon, and dipyridamole may cause increased antiretroviral activity as seen in vitro. Methadone decreases the metabolism. Phenytoin levels can be increased or decreased. Probenecid increases serum concentrations of ZDV.

Important Points: Patients need to take with food. Early side effects may abate over the first month.

Cost: 100 mg capsules No.100 $144.23; $259.61/month maximum dosing.

VACCINES

INFLUENZA VACCINE

Brand Name: Fluogen, Flu-Shield, Fluzone, Flu-Imune.
Class: Vaccine, viral.
Dosage Forms: 5 ml sterile vial, 0.5 ml 1 ml sterile syringes and Tubex.
Indications: Active immunization to influenza virus containing antigens related to those in the vaccine. Recommended for those who wish to reduce the risk of influenza infection. Recommended for infants > 6 months old who are at risk for complications and healthcare workers and others (household contacts) in close contact with patients at risk for development of complications of influenza infection. Patients at risk include:

1. Persons > 65 years of age
2. Residents of nursing homes or chronic-care facilities with chronic medical conditions
3. Adults and children with chronic pulmonary or cardio-

vascular disorders, or children with asthma
4. Adults and children who have previously required regular follow-up or hospitalizations for various chronic conditions including metabolic diseases, renal dysfunction, hemoglobinopathies or immunosuppression
5. Children 6 months to 18 years old receiving long-term aspirin therapy (increased risk for Reye's syndrome).

For persons with HIV infection, recent reports suggest that symptoms of influenza virus infection may be prolonged and the risk for complications may be increased for this risk group. Antibody response may be diminished in this population due to the immunosuppressed condition of patients with HIV infection; however, a booster vaccine has not improved the immune response for these individuals.

Dose: Do not give IV. Give IM injections preferably in the deltoid muscles of adults and older children and in the anterolateral aspect of the thigh in infants and young children. Vaccination is desirable in September, October, or November in easily accessible individuals. Children require different doses depending on age:

- Younger than 9 years old, and not previously vaccinated, require 2 doses of vaccine separated by a 1 month interval.
- Older than 12 years require 0.5 ml whole-virus, split-virus, or purified surface antigen.
- Between the ages of 9 and 12 years require 0.5 ml split-virus or purified surface antigen.
- Between 3 and 8 years old require 1 or 2 doses of 0.5 ml split-virus or purified surface antigen only (No. of doses depends on previous vaccination history)
- Infants between 6 and 35 months need 1 or 2 doses of 0.25 ml of split-virus or purified surface antigen only (see above comment).

Side Effects: Uncommon and mild in adults. Most common is a local reaction at the injection site within 1–2 days of vaccination. Systemic reactions include 2 types: (1) Although infrequent include fever and malaise; seen in first-time recipients of vaccination. Seen within 6–12 hours of vaccination and may persist for 1–2 days. (2) Immediate. May be allergic reaction. Wheal and flare response or respiratory signs and symptoms are extremely rare. May result from sensitivity to vaccine component.

Drug Interactions: Inhibition of the clearance of phenytoin, theophylline, and warfarin has been reported, however, further studies failed to demonstrate clinical significance of these interactions.

Important Points: Only split (subvirion) or purified surface antigen vaccines is recommended in children younger than 8 years of age because of the lower potential for causing febrile reactions. People with febrile illness should not be vaccinated until temporary illness abates. May be administered concomitantly with other oral or injectable vaccines in children and adults (pneumococcus, polio, MMR), however, at different injection sites where applicable. Contraindicated in patients with known hypersensitivity to eggs or egg products.

Cost: Fluogen: 1992–93 5 ml vial $44.44, 0.5 ml single dose No.10 $48.95; Flu-Imune: 1992–93 0.5 ml vials No.10 $40.72.

PNEUMOCOCCUS VACCINE, POLYVALENT

Brand Name: Pneumovax 23, Pnu-Immune 23.

Class: Vaccine, bacterial.

Indications: For immunization against pneumococcal pneumonia and bacteremia caused by the types of pneumocci included in the vaccine. Indicated in adults and children with chronic illnesses at risk for complications of pneumococcal disease. Indicated in asymptomatic and symptomatic HIV-infected adults, as well as in HIV-infected children older than 2 years of age. Indicated in special groups of people living in environmental or social settings associated with an identified increased risk of pneumococcal disease or its complications.

Dosage: Do not inject IV. Administer SC or IM in deltoid muscle or lateral midthigh. Inject 0.5 ml once.

Dosage Form: 1 and 5 dose vials and Lederject^R syringes.

Side Effects: Local erythema and induration at injection site < 48 hours duration and occurs within 1–2 days postinjection. Systemic reactions include low-grade fever, rash, and acute arthralgias within 24 hours. Relapsing ITP up to 2–14 days after injection, lasting up to 2 weeks. Parasthesias, Guillain-Barré syndrome and other CNS manifestations have occurred rarely. Rare anaphylactoid reactions.

Drug Interactions: None listed.

Important Points: Do not give a booster injection to previously vaccinated individuals. May induce arthus reactions and other systemic reactions.

Cost: Pneumovax–2.5 ml multidose vial $47.86, 0.5 ml No.5 $53.69, approximately $10.00/dose.

REFERENCES

Sanford JP: *Guide to Antimicrobial Therapy.* Antimicrobial Therapy, Inc., 1993.

Sanford JP et al: *Guide to HIV/AIDS Therapy.* Antimicrobial Therapy, Inc., 1993.

Dennenberg R: *Guide to Gynecological Care of HIV Positive Women.* Essential Medical Information Systems, Inc., 1993.

Drug Facts and Comparisons, 1993. Facts and Comparisons. A Wolters Klumer Company. St. Louis, MO.

Appendix

- 1993 Revised Classification for HIV Infection and Expanded Surveillance Case Definition for AIDS Among Adolescents and Adults
- Classification of HIV Infection in Children Under 13 Years of Age
- Adult HIV/AIDS Confidential Case Report Form
- TMP/SMX Desensitization Protocol
- Patient Instructions for TMP/SMX Desensitization
- Mental Status Examination
- Florida Living Will and Authorization
- Resources for Practitioners and Patients

1993 REVISED CLASSIFICATION FOR HIV INFECTION AND EXPANDED SURVEILLANCE CASE DEFINITION FOR AIDS AMONG ADOLESCENTS AND ADULTS

	Category A	Category B	Category C
	Asymptomatic or persistent general lymphodenopathy (category A includes acute [primary] infection)	Symptomatic; not category A or C conditions	AIDS indicator conditions*
CD4 Cell Categories			
1) ≥ 500/µg	A1	B1	C1
2) 200–499/µg	A2	B2	C2
3) < 200/µg	A3	B3	C3

The shaded cells illustrate the expanded AIDS surveillance case definition.

Conditions included in the 1993 AIDS surveillance case definition:

- Candidiasis of bronchi, trachea, or lungs
- Candidiasis, esophageal
- Cervical cancer, invasive*
- Coccidioidomycosis, disseminated or extrapulmonary
- Cryptococcosis, extrapulmonary
- Cryptosporidiosis, chronic intestinal (> 1 month duration)
- Cytomegalovirus disease (other than liver, spleen, or nodes)
- Cytomegalovirus retinitis (with loss of vision)
- HIV encephalopathy
- Herpes simplex: chronic ulcer(s) (> 1 month duration) or bronchitis, pneumonitis, or esophagitis
- Histoplasmosis, disseminated or extrapulmonary
- Isosporiasis, chronic intestinal (> 1 month duration)
- Kaposi's sarcoma
- Lymphoma, Burkitt's (or equivalent term)

- Lymphoma, immunoblastic (or equivalent term)
- Lymphoma, primary in brain
- *Mycobacterium avium* complex or *M. kansasii,* disseminated or extrapulmonary
- *Mycobacterium tuberculosis,* any site (pulmonary or extrapulmonary)*
- *Mycobacterium,* other species or unidentified species, disseminated or extrapulmonary
- *Pneumocystis carinii* pneumonia
- Pneumonia, recurrent
- Progressive multifocal leukoencephalopathy
- *Salmonella* septicemia, recurrent
- Toxoplasmosis of brain
- Wasting syndrome resulting from HIV infection

---

*Added in the 1993 expansion of the AIDS surveillance case definition. MMWR: Recommendations and Reports. December 18, 1992, vol. 41, Number RR—17.

CLASSIFICATION OF HIV INFECTION IN CHILDREN UNDER 13 YEARS OF AGE

Class P–0   Indeterminate Infection

Perinatally exposed children < 15 months of age who have a positive HIV antibody test but do not fulfill all the diagnostic criteria for HIV infection.

Class P–1   Asymptomatic Individuals–No present or Previous Signs or Symptoms Leading to Classifications in P–2.

Subclass A: Normal immune function (based on lab data). No immune abnormality associated with HIV infection.
Subclass B: Abnormal immune function (based on lab data), unexplained.
Subclass C: Immune function tests incomplete or not done.

Class P–2   Symptomatic Infection

Subclass A: Nonspecific findings: ≥ 2 findings persisting > 2 months

1. Fever
2. Failure to thrive or weight loss > 10% baseline
3. Hepatomegaly
4. Splenomegaly
5. Generalized lymphadenopathy: ≥ 0.5 cm size, > 2 sites (bilateral nodes count as one site)
6. Parotitis
7. Recurrent or persistent diarrhea: ≥ 2 episodes of ≥ 3 loose stools per day, with dehydration, within a 2 month period.

Subclass B: Progressive Neurologic Disease: At least

one of the following is present:

1. Loss of developmental milestones or intellectual ability
2. Impaired brain growth: acquired microcephaly or brain atrophy demonstrated by CT scan or MRI
3. Progressive symmetrical motor deficits: ≥ 2 of the following:
   a. Paresis
   b. Abnormal tone
   c. Pathologic reflexes
   d. Ataxia
   e. Gait disturbance

Subclass C: Lymphoid Interstitial Pneumonitis.

1. Definitive diagnosis:
   a. Histological confirmation
   b. Diffuse interstitial and peribronchial mononuclear cell infiltrates
   c. No identifiable pathogens
2. Presumptive diagnosis
   a. Bilateral reticulonodular interstitial infiltrates with or without hilar adenopathy on chest radiographs
   b. > 2 months duration
   c. Unresponsive to appropriate antimicrobial therapy
   d. Other causes of interstitial infiltrates excluded

Subclass D: Infectious Diseases.
D–1–Diseases listed in the CDC case definition for AIDS
D–2–Unexplained recurrent serious bacterial infections (≥ 2 in 2 year period)

   a. Sepsis
   b. Meningitis
   c. Pneumonia
   d. Visceral abscess
   e. Bone/joint

D–3–Other infections.

   a. Oral candidiasis of ≥ 2 months duration
   b. Herpes stomatitis ≥ 2 episodes in a 1 year period

    c. Multidermatomal or disseminated herpes zoster
    d. Extra-intestinal strongyloides

Subclass E: Secondary Cancers.
E–1–Malignancies listed in case definition.

    a. Kaposi's sarcoma
    b. B-cell non-Hodgkin's lymphomas
    c. Primary brain lymphoma

E–2–Other malignancies possibly associated with HIV infection.

    a. Other lymphoreticular malignancies
    b. Nasopharyngeal carcinomas

Subclass F: Other Diseases Possibly Resulting from HIV Infection.

1. Hepatitis
2. Cardiomyopathy
3. Nephropathy
4. Hematologic disorders
5. Dermatologic disorders
6. "HIV Embryopathy"

… APPENDIX 207

ADULT HIV/AIDS CONFIDENTIAL CASE REPORT FORM

I. STATE/LOCAL USE ONLY

Patient's Name: _____ (Last, First, M.I.) Phone No.: ( ) _____
Address: _____ City: _____ County: _____ State: _____ Zip Code: _____

RETURN TO STATE/LOCAL HEALTH DEPARTMENT — *Patient identifier information is not transmitted to CDC!* —

U.S. DEPARTMENT OF HEALTH & HUMAN SERVICES
Public Health Service

ADULT HIV/AIDS CONFIDENTIAL CASE REPORT
(Patients ≥13 years of age at time of diagnosis)

CDC

II. HEALTH DEPARTMENT USE ONLY

Form Approved OMB No. 0920-0009

DATE FORM COMPLETED: Mo. __ Day __ Yr. __
SOUNDEX CODE: ____
REPORT STATUS: [1] New Report [2] Update
REPORTING HEALTH DEPARTMENT: State: ____ City: ____ County: ____
State Patient No.: _____
City/County Patient No.: _____
REPORT SOURCE: ____

III. DEMOGRAPHIC INFORMATION

DIAGNOSTIC STATUS AT REPORT (check one):
[1] HIV Infection (not AIDS) — Years ___
[2] AIDS — Years ___

AGE AT DIAGNOSIS: ___

DATE OF BIRTH: Mo. __ Day __ Yr. __

CURRENT STATUS: Alive [1] Dead [2] Unk. [9]

DATE OF DEATH: Mo. __ Day __ Yr. __

STATE/TERRITORY OF DEATH: ____

SEX:
[1] Male
[2] Female

RACE/ETHNICITY:
[1] White (not Hispanic) [2] Black (not Hispanic) [3] Hispanic [4] Asian/Pacific Islander [5] American Indian/Alaska Native [9] Not Specified

COUNTRY OF BIRTH:
[1] U.S. [7] U.S. Dependencies and Possessions (including Puerto Rico) (specify): _____
[8] Other (specify): _____ [9] Unknown

RESIDENCE AT DIAGNOSIS: City: ____ County: ____ State/Country: ____ Zip Code: ____

IV. FACILITY OF DIAGNOSIS

Facility Name: _____
City: _____
State/Country: _____

FACILITY SETTING (check one): [1] Public [2] Private [3] Federal [9] Unknown

FACILITY TYPE (check one): [01] Physician, HMO [31] Hospital, Inpatient [88] Other (specify): _____

This report is authorized by law (Sections 304 and 306 of the Public Health Service Act, 42 USC 242b and 242k). Response in this case is voluntary for federal government purposes, but may be mandatory under state and local statutes. Your cooperation is necessary for the understanding and control of HIV/AIDS. Information in the surveillance system that would permit identification of any individual on whom a record is maintained, is collected with a guarantee that it will be held in confidence, will be used only for the purposes stated in the assurance on file at the local health department, and will not otherwise be disclosed or released without the consent of the individual in accordance with Section 308(d) of the Public Health Service Act (42 USC 242m).

V. PATIENT HISTORY

AFTER 1977 AND PRECEDING THE FIRST POSITIVE HIV ANTIBODY TEST OR AIDS DIAGNOSIS, THIS PATIENT HAD (Respond to ALL Categories):

	Yes	No	Unk.
• Sex with male	1	0	9
• Sex with female	1	0	9
• Injected nonprescription drugs	1	0	9
• Received clotting factor for hemophilia/coagulation disorder	1	0	9

Specify disorder: [1] Factor VIII (Hemophilia A) [2] Factor IX (Hemophilia B) [8] Other (specify): _____

• *HETEROSEXUAL* relations with any of the following:

	Yes	No	Unk.
• Intravenous/injection drug user	1	0	9
• Bisexual male	1	0	9
• Person with hemophilia/coagulation disorder	1	0	9
• Transfusion recipient with documented HIV infection	1	0	9
• Transplant recipient with documented HIV infection	1	0	9
• Person with AIDS or documented HIV infection, risk not specified	1	0	9
• Received transfusion of blood/blood components (other than clotting factor)	1	0	9

First: Mo. __ Yr. __   Last: Mo. __ Yr. __

	Yes	No	Unk.
• Received transplant of tissue/organs or artificial insemination	1	0	9
• Worked in a health-care or clinical laboratory setting	1	0	9

(specify occupation): _____

VI. LABORATORY DATA

1. HIV ANTIBODY TESTS AT DIAGNOSIS: (Indicate first test)

	Pos	Neg	Ind	Not Done	TEST DATE Mo. Yr.
• HIV-1 EIA	1	0	–	9	
• HIV-1/HIV-2 combination EIA	1	0	–	9	
• HIV-1 Western blot/IFA	1	0	8	9	
• Other HIV antibody test (specify):	1	0	8	9	
• HIV-2 EIA	1	0	–	9	
• HIV-2 Western blot	1	0	8	9	

2. POSITIVE HIV DETECTION TEST: (Record earliest test) Mo. __ Yr. __
• HIV culture
• HIV antigen test
• HIV PCR, DNA or RNA probe
• Other (specify): _____

• Date of last documented *negative* HIV test (specify type): _____ Mo. __ Yr. __

• If HIV laboratory tests were not documented, is HIV diagnosis documented by a physician? Yes [1] No [0] Unk. [9]

If yes, provide date of documentation by physician. Mo. __ Yr. __

3. IMMUNOLOGIC LAB TESTS:
AT OR CLOSEST TO CURRENT DIAGNOSTIC STATUS   Mo. __ Yr. __
• CD4 Count _____ cells/μL
• CD4 Percent _____ %

First <200 μL or <14%   Mo. __ Yr. __
• CD4 Count _____ cells/μL
• CD4 Percent _____ %

CDC 50.42A REV. 07-93 (Page 1 of 2) – ADULT HIV/AIDS CONFIDENTIAL CASE REPORT –

208 APPENDIX

VII. STATE/LOCAL USE ONLY

Physician's Name: _____ Phone No.: ( ) _____ Medical Record No. _____
(Last, First, M.I.)
Hospital/Facility: _____ Person Completing Form: _____ Phone No.: ( ) _____

– *Physician identifier information is not transmitted to CDC!* –

VIII. CLINICAL STATUS

CLINICAL RECORD REVIEWED:	Yes [1]	No [0]	ENTER DATE PATIENT WAS DIAGNOSED AS:	Asymptomatic (including acute retroviral syndrome and persistent generalized lymphadenopathy): Mo. Yr.		Symptomatic (not AIDS): Mo. Yr.

AIDS INDICATOR DISEASES	Initial Diagnosis Def. Pres.	Initial Date Mo. Yr.	AIDS INDICATOR DISEASES	Initial Diagnosis Def. Pres.	Initial Date Mo. Yr.
Candidiasis, bronchi, trachea, or lungs	[1] NA		Lymphoma, Burkitt's (or equivalent term)	[1] NA	
Candidiasis, esophageal	[1] [2]		Lymphoma, immunoblastic (or equivalent term)	[1] NA	
Carcinoma, invasive cervical	[1] NA		Lymphoma, primary in brain	[1] NA	
Coccidioidomycosis, disseminated or extrapulmonary	[1] NA		*Mycobacterium avium* complex or *M.kansasii*, disseminated or extrapulmonary	[1] [2]	
Cryptococcosis, extrapulmonary	[1] NA		*M. tuberculosis*, pulmonary*	[1] [2]	
Cryptosporidiosis, chronic intestinal (>1 mo. duration)	[1] NA		*M. tuberculosis*, disseminated or extrapulmonary*	[1] [2]	
Cytomegalovirus disease (other than in liver, spleen, or nodes)	[1] NA		*Mycobacterium*, of other species or unidentified species, disseminated or extrapulmonary	[1] [2]	
Cytomegalovirus retinitis (with loss of vision)	[1] [2]		*Pneumocystis carinii* pneumonia	[1] [2]	
HIV encephalopathy	[1] NA		Pneumonia, recurrent, in 12 mo. period	[1] [2]	
Herpes simplex: chronic ulcer(s) (>1 mo. duration); or bronchitis, pneumonitis or esophagitis	[1] NA		Progressive multifocal leukoencephalopathy	[1] NA	
Histoplasmosis, disseminated or extrapulmonary	[1] NA		Salmonella septicemia, recurrent	[1] NA	
Isosporiasis, chronic intestinal (>1 mo. duration)	[1] NA		Toxoplasmosis of brain	[1] [2]	
Kaposi's sarcoma	[1] [2]		Wasting syndrome due to HIV	[1] NA	

Def. = definitive diagnosis   Pres. = presumptive diagnosis   * RVCT CASE NO.: _____

• If HIV tests were not positive or were not done, does this patient have an immunodeficiency that would disqualify him/her from the AIDS case definition?   [1] Yes   [0] No   [9] Unknown

IX. TREATMENT/SERVICES REFERRALS

Has this patient been informed of his/her HIV infection?   [1] Yes   [0] No   [9] Unk.

This patient's partners will be notified about their HIV exposure and counseled by:
[1] Health department   [2] Physician/provider   [3] Patient   [9] Unknown

This patient is receiving or has been referred for:
	Yes	No	NA	Unk.
• HIV related medical services	[1]	[0]	–	[9]
• Substance abuse treatment services	[1]	[0]	[8]	[9]

This patient received or is receiving:
• Anti-retroviral therapy .... Yes [1] No [0] Unk. [9]
• PCP prophylaxis .... Yes [1] No [0] Unk. [9]

This patient has been enrolled at:
Clinical Trial: [1] NIH-sponsored [2] Other [3] None [9] Unknown
Clinic: [1] HRSA-sponsored [2] Other [3] None [9] Unknown

This patient's medical treatment is *primarily* reimbursed by:
[1] Medicaid   [2] Private insurance/HMO   [3] No coverage   [4] Other Public Funding   [7] Clinical trial/government program   [9] Unknown

FOR WOMEN:
• This patient is receiving or has been referred for gynecological or obstetrical services: .... [1] Yes   [0] No   [9] Unknown
• Is this patient currently pregnant? .... [1] Yes   [0] No   [9] Unknown
• Has this patient delivered live-born infants? .... [1] Yes (if delivered after 1977, provide birth information below for the most recent birth)   [0] No   [9] Unknown

CHILD'S DATE OF BIRTH: Mo. __ Day __ Yr. __   Hospital of Birth: _____   City: _____   State: _____   **Child's Soundex:** _____   **Child's State Patient No.:** _____

X. COMMENTS: _____

Public burden for this collection of information is estimated to average 10 minutes per response. Send comments regarding this burden estimate or any other aspect of this collection of information, including suggestions for reducing this burden to PHS Reports Clearance Officer; ATTN: PRA; Hubert H. Humphrey Bg, Rm 721-B; 200 Independence Ave., SW; Washington, DC 20201, and to the Office of Management and Budget; Paperwork Reduction Project (0920-0009); Washington, DC 20503. – **DO NOT MAIL CASE REPORT FORMS TO THESE ADDRESSES** –

CDC 50.42A REV. 07-93 (Page 2 of 2)   – ADULT HIV/AIDS CONFIDENTIAL CASE REPORT –

TMP/SMX DESENSITIZATION PROTOCOL

TMP/SMX is the drug of choice for PCP prophylaxis. In addition there is evidence that TMP/SMX also may prevent the development of toxoplasmosis encephalitis. Unfortunately, some 25% of HIV-infected persons have allergic reactions to TMP/SMX. Several studies with various desensitization protocols have reported upwards of 50% success rates. Patients chosen to try desensitization should be screened carefully and those with a history of a severe reaction or generalized body rash should not be selected. Patients should be informed of allergic symptoms and signs and closely followed during the desensitization process.

Other protocols exist for sulfadiazine and dapsone desensitization.

Physician Instructions

1. Write prescriptions for the following:
    a. TMP/SMX Pediatric oral suspension–No.30 cc
       Sig: Use as directed
    b. TMP/SMX DS No.30
       Sig: Use as directed
    c. Sterile water–20 cc
       Sig: Use as directed
    d. Diphenhydramine 25 mg
       Sig: i-ii tabs PO TID prn itching or rash.
2. Give PATIENT INSTRUCTION SHEET (see following page).
3. Give patient 1 cc syringe and 10 cc syringe.

REFERENCES

Carr A et al: Low-dose trimethoprim-sulfasoxazole prophylaxis for toxoplasmic encephalitis in patients with AIDS. *Ann Int Med* 1992;**117**:106.

Carr A, Penny R, Cooper D: Efficacy and safety of rechallenge with low-dose trimethoprim-sulfamethoxazole in previously hypersensitive HIV-infected patients. *AIDS* 1993;**7**:65.

Shafer RW, Seitzman PA, Tapper ML: Successful prophylaxis of *Pneumocystis carinii* pneumonia with trimethoprim-sulfamethoxazole in AIDS patients with previous allergic reactions. *J AIDS* 1989;**2(4):**389.

White MV et al: Desensitization to trimethoprim sulfamethoxazole in patients with acquired immune deficiency syndrome and *Pneumocystis carinii* pneumonia. *Ann Allergy* 1989;**62:**177.

PATIENT INSTRUCTIONS FOR TMP/SMX DESENSITIZATION

1. Label your medicine as follows:
   A = Sterile water bottle 20 cc
   B = TMP/SMX Pediatric suspension
   C = TMP/SMX DS tabs
2. Carefully open Bottle A. Do not throw away the rubber stopper. Using the 1 cc syringe, remove 1 cc of water from the bottle and discard it. Using the same syringe, transfer 1 cc from Bottle B to Bottle A. Bottle A now contains a 1:20 dilution of medicine B.
3. Use medicine A on days 1–4.
   Use medicine B on days 5–9.
   Use medicine C on days 10–18.

Day	Medication	Amount
1	A	1.0 cc
2	A	2.0 cc
3	A	4.0 cc
4	A	8.0 cc
5	B	0.6 cc
6	B	1.25 cc
7	B	2.5 cc
8	B	5.0 cc
9	B	10 cc
10	C	1/2 tab once daily
11	C	1/2 tab twice daily
12	C	1/2 tab twice daily
13	C	1/2 tab twice daily
14	C	1/2 tab twice daily
15	C	1/2 tab twice daily
16	C	1/2 tab twice daily
17	C	1/2 tab twice daily
18	C	1 whole tablet once daily

Notify a physician immediately if you experience any itching, rash, shortness of breath, nausea, vomiting, diarrhea, fever, or any other unusual symptoms.

MENTAL STATUS EXAMINATION

The Short Blessed Test*

	Maximum Error	Score	Weight	Total
1. What year is it now?	1 wrong	____	x 4 =	____
2. What month is it now? Repeat the following memory phrase: "John Brown, 42 Market Street, Chicago"	1 wrong	____	x 3 =	____
3. What time is it? (within 1 hour is correct)	1 wrong	____	x 3 =	____
4. Count backwards 20 to 1.	2 wrong	____	x 2 =	____
5. Say the months in reverse order.	2 wrong	____	x 2 =	____
6. Repeat memory phrase from above: (omitting "street" is not counted as an error)	5 wrong	____	x 2 =	____

Total Score: _____

Scoring:

≤ 8	normal or minimal impairment
9–19	moderate impairment
≥ 20	severe impairment

From *Am J Psych* 1983;**140**:739. Copyright 1983, The American Psychiatric Association. Reprinted with permission.

REFERENCES

Katzman R et al: Validation of a short orientation-memory-concentration test of cognitive impairment. *Am J Psych* 1983;**140:**734.

Davis P et al: Brief screening tests versus clinical staging in senile dementia of the Alzheimer type. *J Am Geriatrics Society* 1990;**38:**129.

FLORIDA LIVING WILL AND AUTHORIZATION

Declaration made this _____ day of _____, 19____.

I_____, willfully and voluntarily make known my desire that my dying not be artificially prolonged under the circumstances set forth below, and I do hereby declare:

If at any time I should have a terminal condition and if my attending physician has determined that there can be no recovery from such condition and that my death is imminent, I direct that life-prolonging procedures be withheld or withdrawn when the application of such procedures would serve only to prolong artificially the process of dying and that I be permitted to die naturally with only the administration of medication or the performance of any medical procedure deemed necessary to provide me with comfort care or to alleviate pain. I do ( ) I do not ( ) desire that nutrition and hydration (food and water) be held or withdrawn when the application of such procedures would serve only to prolong artificially the process of dying.

In the event that I am comatose or otherwise mentally or physically incapable of personally declaring my intentions, I authorize:

_____

(Print Name)

who is: ( ) my health care surrogate, ( ) my attorney-in-fact, ( ) other _____ (specify) to make decisions for me concerning the witholding or withdrawal of life-prolonging procedures.

In the absence of my ability to give directions regarding the use of such life-prolonging procedures, it is my intention that this declaration be honored by my family and physician as the final expression of my legal right to refuse medical or surgical treatment and to accept the consequences for such refusal.

I understand the full import of this declaration, and I am emotionally and mentally competent to make this declaration.

_____

DECLARANT

The declarant is known to me and I believe him or her to be of sound mind and under no duress, fraud or undue influence.

_____ _____ WITNESS

_____ _____ (Print Name)

_____
(Address and Telephone Number)

_____ _____ WITNESS

_____ _____ (Print Name)

_____
(Address and Telephone Number)

Contact Hospice Link: 800-331-1620 for information about Living Wills in your state.

RESOURCES FOR PRACTITIONERS AND PATIENTS

General Information

National AIDS/HIV Hotline
  English: 800-342-2437 (24 hours)
  Spanish: 800-344-7432 (8 AM–2 PM Eastern time, Monday–Friday)
  Hearing impaired: 800-243-7889 (10 AM–10 PM Eastern time)
National AIDS Information Clearinghouse: 800-458-5231
American Foundation for AIDS Research (AmFar): 800-392-6327
Gay Men's Health Crisis AIDS Hotline: 212-807-6655
Project Inform: 800-822-7422
AIDS Treatment Data Network: 212-268-4196
National Pediatric HIV Resource Center: 800-362-0071
National Association of People with AIDS: 202-898-0414
Teens Teaching AIDS Prevention Program: 800-234-8336

Clinical Trials

AIDS Clinical Trials Information Service: 800-TRIALS-A (9 AM–7 PM Eastern time, Monday–Friday)
National Institutes of Health AIDS Trials: 800-243-7644
Community Research Initiative on AIDS: 212-924-3934

Education for Physicians/Practitioners

HIV Telephone Consultation Service for Health Care Providers 800-933-3413 (7:30 AM–5 PM Pacific time, Monday–Friday)

AIDS Education and Training Centers

New York/Virgin Islands: 212-305-3616
Washington, Alaska, Montana, Idaho, Oregon: 206-720-4250
Ohio, Michigan, Kentucky, Tennessee: 614-292-1400
Nevada, Arizona, Hawaii, California (north): 209-252-2851
Southern California: 213-342-1846
Southern Alabama, Georgia, North Carolina, South Carolina: 404-727-2929
Arkansas, Louisiana, Mississippi: 504-568-3855
North and South Dakota, Utah, Colorado, New Mexico, Nebraska, Kansas, Wyoming: 303-355-1301
Iowa, Minnesota, Wisconsin, Illinois, Indiana, Missouri: 312-966-1373
W. Virginia, Delaware, Virginia, Maryland: 804-786-2210
Connecticut, Maine, Massachusetts, New Hampshire, Rhode Island, Vermont: 508-856-3255
Texas, Oklahoma: 713-794-4075
Pennsylvania: 412-624-1895
New Jersey: 201-982-3690
Florida: 305-585-7836
Puerto Rico: 809-759-6528
Washington, DC area: 202-865-6249

Journals/Newsletters

AIDS Clinical Care (monthly): 800-843-6356
AIDS Treatment News: 800-873-2812
BETA: Bulletin of Experimental Treatments for AIDS: 800-327-9893
PWA Newsline: 800-828-3280
Treatment Issues: 212-337-3695
The Positive Woman: 202-898-0372
Physicians Association for AIDS Care (PAAC) News: 312-222-1326

Pharmaceutical Information

Selected Buyers' Clubs for AIDS drugs: (see Chapter 13 for more information)
    Carl Vogel Foundation: 202-289-4898
    Healing Alternatives Foundation: 415-626-2316
    PWA Health Group 212-255-0520
    PWA Health Link 1-800-456-4792

Selected Payment Assistance Programs and Expanded Access Programs

Acyclovir; atovaquone; pyrimethamine; TMP/SMX; zidovudine(Burroughs-Wellcome): 800-772-9294
Alfa-Interferon-2a, zalcitabine (Hoffman-LaRoche): 800-443-6676
Alfa-Interferon-2b (Schering-Plough): 800-521-7157
Azithromycin (Pfizer): 800-742-3029
Ciprofloxacin (Miles): 800-998-9180
Clarithromycin (Abbott): 800-688-9118
Didanosine, Megestrol (Bristol-Myers-Squibb): 800-788-0123
Dronabinol (Roxane): 800-274-8651
Erythropoetin (Ortho Biotech): 800-553-3851
Filgrastim (Amgen): 800-272-9376
Fluconazole (Pfizer): 800-869-9979
Foscarnet (Astra): 800-488-3247
Ganciclovir (Syntex): 800-444-4200
Itraconazole (Janssen): 800-544-2987
Liposomal Daunorubicin (Vestar): 800-247-3303
Octreotide acetate (Sandoz): 800-447-6673
Pentamidine (Fujisawa): 800-366-6323
Rifabutin (Adria): 800-795-9759
Streptomycin (Pfizer) 800-254-4445
Trimetrexate (US Bioscience) 800-8US BIOS

Index

Abdominal pain, causes of, 52–53
Acid fast bacilli (AFB)
    isolation, comparison of with respiratory isolation, 76
    staining and culture, 71
Acquired immunodeficiency syndrome (AIDS), epidemic. *See also* HIV infection
    education and training centers, 217
    reporting requirements by state, 3
    trends in United States, 1–3,
    wasting syndrome, drugs for, 170, 180
ACTG
    076 clinical trial, 114
    114 clinical trial, 39
Acyclovir, for herpes, 29, 91, 160
    topical, 1612
Adolescents
    number of AIDs cases associated with, 2
    pretest counseling for, 6–7
    revised classification for HIV infection and expanded surveillance case definition for AIDs among, 202–203
Adult HIV/AIDS Confidential case report form, 207–208
Adults, revised classification for HIV infection and expanded surveillance case definition for AIDs among, 202–203
AFB. *See* Acid fast bacilli
Age
    Age/CD4 criteria for PCP prophylaxis, 126
    ranges, and number of AIDs cases, 2
AIDS. *See* Acquired immunodeficiency syndrome
Alfa-interferon 2A and 2B, 161–162
Alkabam-AQ, 195–196
Alpha-fetoprotein and amniocentesis, 113
Alternative medical practices and AIDs, 148. *See also* Experimental and nontraditional treatments for AIDs
Amebiasis, drugs for, 185
Amenorrhea in HIV-infected women, 111
Amikacin, 162–163
Amikin, 162
Amniocentesis and alpha–fetoprotein, 113
Amphotericin, for *Cryptococcus,* 51
    Amphotericin B, 163–164
    for meningitis, 49
Anabolic agents, as nutritional supplementation, 139–140
Anaerobic infections, drugs for, 181

INDEX

Anemia
  in HIV patient, 19–20
  from zidovudine use, 124
Anergic patients, 72
Anorexia, nutritional issues, 140
Antioxidants, as nutritional supplementation, 138–139
Antiretroviral agents (in children), 127–129
  didanosine, 128–129
  indications, 127
  zidovudine, 128
Antiretroviral therapy and strategy, 21, 34–40, 41–44
  considerations in evaluation of, 20–21
  didanosine, 36
  discontinuing, 43–44
  failure, 42–43
  naive patients, 42
  sequence, 43
  stavudine, 39–40
  zalcitabine, 38–39
  zidovudine (ZDV), 34–36
Antiretrovirals, drugs for, 192, 196
Antiviral therapy for pregnant HIV–infected woman, 114
Appetite stimulants, 139
Aspergillus, drugs for, 177
Asymptomatic children, and frequency of follow-up, 125
Atovaquone, 164
Azithromycin, 165
AZT. *See* Zidovudine

B_{12} injections, 138
Bactrim, 193–194
  Bactrim DS, 193–194
  for *Pneumocystis carinii*, 24
Beta–carotene, 138
$beta_2$ microglobulin test, 15
Biaxin, 165–166
Bisexual men, number of AIDs cases associated with, 1
Blacks, number of AIDs cases among, 2
Blood and bloody secretions, precautions for handling, 123
Body composition analysis and anthropometrics, 135–136
Buyer's clubs for AIDs drugs, 148–149

Candida antigen, 70
Candidiasis
  diagnosis, 46
  drugs for, 163, 173, 177, 178, 183, 191
  other *Candida* infections, 47
  presentation, 45–46
  treatment, 46–47
Care for HIV infection
  essential pathophysiology and medical management of, 12
  key components of, 11
CD4 cell count
  below age–related criteria, 127
  calculation of absolute, 22
  criteria for PCP prophylaxis, 126
  evaluation of count, 20–21
  low, 43
  patients with over 500, 34
  range of in children, 124–125
  receptor interpretation, 12
Centers for Disease Control (CDC)
  AIDs cases reported to, 2, 13
  expansion of definition of AIDs, 63
  voluntary surveillance project for health care workers with occupational HIV exposure, 154–155
Central nervous system (CNS), cells of, 12
Cervical dysplasia and neoplasia, 111–112
Children, HIV infection in
  antiretroviral agents, 127–129
  common pediatric HIV-associated infections and conditions, 129–131
  comprehensive and anticipatory health maintenance, 123–124
  follow-up examination, 124–125
  health maintenance, 122–123
  other therapies, 129
  Pneumocystis carinii pneumonia prophylaxis, 125–126
  screening of infants born to seropositive women, 121–122
  testing considerations, 120–121
  under 13 years of age, classification of HIV infection in, 204–206
Chorioretinitis, 55
Ciprofloxacin, 189–190
Clarithromycin, 26, 35, 165–166

Cleocin, 166
Clindamycin, 166
Clinical trials for AIDs, 216
Clofazamine, 26, 166–167
Clotrimazole
   cream, 167–168
   troche, 167
CMV. *See* Cytomegalovirus
Coccidiomycosis immitis, 28
   diagnosis, 48–49
   drugs for, 173
   presentation, 47–48
   treatment, 49
Community resources for HIV patient, exploring, 17
Community Programs for Clinical Research on AIDs (CPCRA), 147
Copper deficiencies, 138
Counseling for HIV infection
   for adolescents, 6–7
   posttest counseling, 8–9
   pretest counseling, 6–7
CPCRA 002 trial, 39
Cryptococcus infection, drugs for, 163, 173, 177
Cryptococcus neoformans, 28
   diagnosis, 51
   presentation, 50–51
   treatment, 51–52
Cryptosporidium, 52–53
   treatment, 53
Cytomegalovirus (CMV), 20, 54–57
   diagnosis, 55–56
   drugs for, 174, 175
   presentation, 54–55
   recommendation, 29
   prophylaxis, 29
   treatment, 56–57
Cystosine arabinoside, IV and intrathecal, 82
Cytovene, 175–176

D4T. *See* Stavudine
Dapsone, 168
   for *Pneumocystis carinii*, 24
Daraprim, 188
ddC. *See* Zalcitabine
ddI. *See* Didanosine
Depression
   drugs for, 180

   nutritional issues, 142
Dermatological manifestations in HIV-infected individuals, 93
   complaints, 93
   diagnostic approaches to, 95–98
Diarrhea
   causes of, 52–53
   drugs for, 169, 179, 184
   in HIV-infected persons, 93, 99
   nutritional issues, 140
Didanosine, 36, 114, 168–169
   dosage, 37, 129
   indications, 36–37, 129
   monitoring, 38
   toxicity and side effects, 37–38, 129
Diet history analysis, as part of nutritional status assessment, 135
Differential diagnosis of common complaints in HIV-infected persons. *See* specific complaints
Diflucan, 173–174
Diphenoxylate with Atropine, 169–170
Disease-related complications and nutritional issues, 140–142
Dronabinol, 170
Drug susceptibility testing, 71
Drugs. *See* Medications; specific medications
Drugs for AIDs, experimental and unlicensed, 148–149. *See also* Experimental and nontraditional treatments for AIDs
Dysphagia
   of HIV-infected persons, 94, 104
   nutritional issues, 140
Dyspnea, nutritional issues, 140

Education centers for AIDs, 217
Elevated liver enzymes, in HIV-infected person, 94, 102
Enoxacin, 189–190
Enteral and parenteral nutrition in HIV patients, 143
Enzyme-linked immunosorbent assay (ELISA) HIV antibody test, 8
Epidemic. *See* Acquired immunodeficiency syndrome
Epogen, 170–172
Epstein-Barr virus, drugs for, 160

Erythropoietin, epoetin alfa, EPO, 170–172
Esophageal candida, 46
  diagnosis, 46
  presentation, 45
  treatment, 46–47
Ethambutol, 172
Examination, follow-up. *See* Follow-up examination
Experimental and nontraditional treatments for AIDs, 147–149

False-positive results of HIV testing, 8
Fat malabsorption, nutritional issues, 141
Fatigue
  as common complaint of HIV-infected persons, 94, 100
  severe, drugs for, 180
Ferritin, 136
Fever
  HIV-infected person with, 94, 101
  nutritional issues, 142
Filgrastim, 172–173
Flagyl, 181–182
Flint SSD, 191–192
Flu-Immune, 197–199
Flu-Shield, 197–199
Fluconazole, 173–174
Fluogen, 197–199
Fluzone, 197–199
Focal neurologic findings in HIV-infected persons, 103
Folinic acid, 174
Follow-up examination
  CD4 count, calculation, 22
  frequency, 21–22
  interval history, 19
  laboratory results, 19–21
  physical examination, 19
  systems review, 19
Foscarnet, 56, 174–175
Foscavir, 174–175
Fungal infections, medications for, 28
Fungal prophylaxis, 28
  recommendations, 28
Fungizone, 163–164
Fungus infections, drugs for, 167, 168, 178, 179

Gallium scan, 79
Ganciclovir, 56, 175–176
Gardnerella vaginalis, drugs for, 181
Gastrointestinal disease, 55
Gastrointestinal (GI) tract, cells of, 12
Genital lesions, 58
GI disease. *See* Gastrontestnal disease
Gynecological concerns of HIV-infected women, 107–108

Haemophilis influenzae type b
  type b virus, of children, 122
  vaccine for HIV patient, 16
Hairy leukoplakia, drugs for, 160
Headaches of HIV-infected persons, 94, 103
Health care workers and occupational exposure to HIV, 151–155
  HIV-infected workers, 155
  post-exposure zidovudine, 153–155
  recommendations, 152–153
  universal precautions, 152–153
Health maintenance, 16–17, 122–123
  of children, comprehensive and anticipatory, 123–124
  of children, immunizations, 122
Hepatitis B vaccine
  for children, 122
  for HIV patient, 16
Hepatomegaly of HIV-infected persons, 94, 102
Herpes simplex, 57–59
  acycolvir-resistant, 174, 175
  diagnosis, 58–59
  drugs for, 160, 161
  presentation, 58
  prophylaxis, 29
  recommendations, 29
  treatment, 59
Heterosexuals, number of AIDs cases associated with, 1
Hispanics, number of AIDs cases among, 2
Histoplasmosis, 60–61
  diagnosis, 60–61
  drugs for, 177
  presentation, 60
  treatment, 61
HIV infection
  antibody test, 124

INDEX

cardiomyopathy in children, 131
care. *See* Care for HIV
culture/PCR/p24 antigen, 124
encephalopathy in children, 131
nephropathy in children, 131
reporting requirements by state, 3
risk of to health care workers 155.
  See also Health care workers
testing. *See* Testing
HIV-1 infection, 8
HIV-2 infection, 8
Hivid, 38–39, 196. *See* Zalcitabine
Homosexual men, number of AIDs cases associated with,1
Humatin, 185
Hyperamylasemia, 38

IDU. *See* Injecting drug use
Immune system function, preservation, 11, 12
Immunizations needed for HIV patient, 16–17
Imodium and Imodium-AD, 179–180
Indirect immunofluorescent assay (IFA), 8
Infants born to seropositive women, screening, 121–122
  examination, 121
  history, 121
  laboratory, 121–122
Infections of HIV-infected women, gynecological, 108–111
  Candida vaginitis, 108
  common HIV. *See* specific infections
Infections, common pediatric HIV-associated, 129–131
Influenza vaccine, for HIV patient, 16, 197–199
INH
  with pyridoxime, 73
  with rifampin, 73
Injecting drug-use (IDU), AIDs cases associated with, 1
Intrapartum considerations of HIV-infected pregnant woman, 115–116
2b-Intron A, 161–162
Isoniazid, 176–177
Isospora belli, 52–53
  treatment, 53–54

ITP. *See* Thrombocytopenia
Itraconazole, for Candida, 47, 177
IV immune globulin (IVIG), 129

Journals and newsletters, AIDs, 217

Kaposi's Sarcoma (KS), 61–63
  diagnosis, 62
  drugs for, 195
  presentation, 61–62
  treatment, 62–63
Ketoconazole, 178–179
  cream, 179
  for *Candida*, 47
KS. *See* Kaposi's sarcoma

Laboratory tests taken for initial visit for HIV patient, 15
Laboratory results, interpretation, 19–21
  anemia, CBC, 19–20
  CD4 cells, 20–21
  leukopenia, differential, 20
  renal function, chemistry, 20
  thrombocytopenia, platelets, 20
  PPD, 20
Laboratory results of HIVinfected child, interpretation
  CD4 cells, 124–125
  HIV culture, 124
  quantitative immunoglobulins, 125
Lamprene, 166–167
Laniazid, 176
Lesions of KS, local, 62–63
Leucovorin, 174
Leukopenia, in HIV patient, 20
Liver enzymes, elevated, in HIV-infected person, 94, 102
Liver function tests, 75
Living will and authorization, Florida, 214–215
Lofene, 169–170
Lomefloxacin, 189–190
Lomodix, 169–170
Lomonate, 169–170
Lomotil, 169–170
Lonox, 169–170
Loperamide, 179
Lotrimin, 167–168
Low-Quel, 169–170

Lumbar puncture, for *Cryptococcus*, 51
Lymphoid interstitial pneumonitis, in children, 130
　diagnosis, 130
　presentation, 130
　treatment, 130
Lymphoma, HIV-related, 63–65
　diagnosis, 64–65
　presentation, 64
　treatment, 65

MAC. *See Mycobacterium avium* complex
MAI. *See Mycobacterium avium* complex
Malnutrition, risk of, 133–134. *See also* Nutrition
Marinol, 170
Measles serostatus for children, 122
Medical history of HIV patient, taking, 13
Medical management of HIV infection, 12
Medication index for HIV-infected individuals, 158–159
Medications for HIV-infected individuals
　index, 158–159
　medications, 160–197. *See also* specific medications
　resources, 157–158
　vaccines, 159–160, 197–200
Medium Chain Triglyceride oil, 141
Megace, 180
Megestrol acetate, 180
Men, ages 25–44, HIV as leading cause of death in, 2
Meningitis, treatment of, 49
Menstrual disorders of HIV-infected women, 111
Mental status examination, 212
Mepron, 164
Methylphenidate, 180–181
Metronidazole, 181–182
Microsporida, 52–53
　treatment, 54
Minerals, as nutritional supplementation, 138
MMR, for HIV patient, 16
Morphine sulfate continuous release, 182–183

MS Contin, 182
MTB. *See Mycobacterium tuberculosis*
Multiple drug–resistant MTB (MDRTB), 69
　among children and adults, 73
　exposure to, 72
　recommendations, 74
Myambutol, 172
Mycelex, 167–168
　Troche, 167
Mycobacterium avium complex (MAC), 19, 65–67
　diagnosis, 66
　drugs for, 161, 165, 166, 172, 189, 190, 191
　indications for prophylaxis, 26
　medications for, 25–27
　presentation, 66
　prophylaxis, 67, 126
　Rifabutin, 26–27
　treatment, 66–67
　under investigation, 26
　zidovudine, 27
Mycobacterium tuberculosis (MTB), 19–20, 69–77
　diagnosis, 70–71
　drugs for, 161, 172, 176, 187, 190, 191, 192
　multiple drug-resistant, 69
　presentation, 67–68
　prevention and control, 75–77
　treatment, 71–75
Mycobutin, 190
Mycostatin, 183
Myopathy, 35
Myositis, 35

National Behavioral Surveys (NABS), and HIV testing, 5
National Institute of Allergy and Infectious Diseases (NIAID)
　AIDS Clinical Trial Group (ACTG), 147
　recommendations on retroviral therapy, 41
Nebupent, 186
Neoplasia and cervical dysplasia, 111–112
Neupogen, 172–173
Neurologic disease, 55, 56
Neurologic findings of HIV-infected persons, 94, 103

INDEX

Neurosyphilis, 83, 84
Neutrexin, 194–195
Neutropenia, 35
Nilstat, 183
Nizoral, 178–179
Non-Hodgkins lymphoma, 63
Nontraditional treatments for AIDS, 147–149
Norfloxacin, 189–190
Normocytic anemia, 35
Nutrient supplementation/augmentation, recommended, 137–140
Nutrition as essential component in care of HIV-infected individual, 16
   common disease-related complications and issues, 140–142
   components of, 135–137
   patterns of wasting and weight loss, 134
   risk of malnutrition, 133–134
   specialized nutrition support, 143
   supplementation/augmentation, 137–140
   women and wasting, 134
Nutritional status assessment, 135–136
   body composition analysis, 135–136
   diet history analysis, 135
   evaluation of biochemical parameters, 136
Nydrazid, 176
Nystatin, 183

O-V Statin, 183
Obstetric sonograms, 113
Occupational exposure to HIV, 151–155
Octreotide, 184
Odynophagia of HIV-infected persons, 94, 104
Ofloxacin, 189–190
Opium, tincture of, 184–185
Opportunistic infection
   during pregnancy, treatment, 115
   prophylaxis in pregnancy, 115
Opportunistic infections, prevention
   cytomegalovirus prophylaxis, 29
   early care for, 11
   fungal prophylaxis, 29
   herpes simplex prophylaxis, 29
   mycobacterium avium complex (MAC) prophylaxis, 25–27
   pneumocystis carinii pneumonia (PCP) prophylaxis, 23–25
   toxoplasmosis encephalitis prophylaxis, 27–28
Oral Candida, 45–46
   diagnosis, 46
   presentations, 45–46
   treatment, 46
Oral acyclovir, for Herpes, 59
Oramorph SR, 182

P-24 antigen, test, 8, 15
Pain, drugs for, 182
Pancreatitis, 38
Paromomycin, 185
Parvovirus, 20
Parenteral and enteral nutrition in HIV patients, 143
Patient follow-up examination. *See* Follow–up examination
Patient visit
   expectations and questions, 14–15
   health maintenance, 16–17
   history, 13
   laboratory test, 15
   past medical history, 13
   physical exam, 15
   psychosocial history, 14
   review of systems, 14
Patients, resources for, 216–218
Payment assistant and expanded access programs, AIDs, 218
PCP. *See Pneumocystis carinii*
Pediatric HIV-associated infections and conditions, therapies for, 129
Pelvic Inflammatory disease (PID), in HIVinfected women, 111
Pentam 300, 185–186
Pentamidine
   inhaled, 186
   IV, 185–186
   for *Pneumocystis carinii,* 25
   PCP prophylaxis, 77
Peripheral neuropathy of HIV-infected persons, 38, 95, 105
Pharmaceutical information, AIDs, 218
Physical examination of HIV patient
   initial, 15
   of HIV patient, on follow-up visit, 19
Physicians, education for, 216
PID. *See* Pelvic inflammatory disease
PML. *See* Progressive multifocal leukoencephalopathy

Pneumococcus vaccine, polyvalent, 199–200
Pneumocystis carinii pneumonia (PCP) prophylaxis, 23–25, 48, 78–80, 125–126
  age/CD4 criteria for, 126
  diagnosis, 79
  diagnosis in children, 130
  drugs for, 164, 166, 185, 186, 187, 194, 195
  indications for primary prophylaxis, 24
  indications for secondary prophylaxis, 24
  medications, 24–25
  pneumonia in children, therapies for, 130
  presentation, 78
  presentation in children, 130
  recommended drug regimen for children older than one month, 126
  regimen choice, 25
  treatment, 79–80
  treatment in children, 130
Pneumonia, 55, 56
Pneumonococcal vaccine for HIV patient, 16
Pneumovax 23, 199–200
Pnu-Immune 23, 199–200
Polymerase chain reaction (PCR), 8
Post-exposure zidovudine in health care workers, 153–155
Postherpetic neuralgia, 92
Postpartum considerations in HIV-infected woman, 116
Posttest counseling for HIV infection, 8–9
PPD for HIV patient, 20
Practitioners
  education for, 216
  resources for, 216–218
Precautions for health care workers, universal, 152–153
Pregnancy in HIV-infected women, 112–116
  antiviral therapy, 114
  effectiveness of methods to prevent, 109–111
  follow-up visit, 113
  intrapartum considerations, 115–116
  opportunistic infection prophylaxis in pregnancy, 115
  postpartum considerations, 116
  prenatal care, initial visit, 112–113
  treatment of opportunistic infections during pregnancy, 115
Prenatal care of HIV-infected woman, initial visit, 112–113
  laboratory, 112–113
  review of systems, 112
Pretest counseling for HIV infection, 6–7
Prevention
  of AIDs, use of HIV test for, 9–10
  of opportunistic infections. *See* Opportunistic infections, prevention
Primaquine, 187
Procrit, 170–172
Progressive cutaneous and disseminated disease, 63
Progressive multifocal leukoencephalopathy, 81–82
  diagnosis, 81
  presentation, 81–82
  treatment, 82
Prophylaxis against opportunistic infection, 11
Protostat, 181–182
Psychologic stress, nutritional issues, 142
Psychosocial assessment of HIV-infected child, 123
Psychosocial history of HIV patent, taking, 14
Pyrazinamide, 187–188
Pyridoxine, 71
Pyrimethamine, 53, 188

Quality of life in HIV patient, optimizing, 11
Quantitative immunoglobulins, 125
Quinolone antibiotics, 37, 189–190

Rectal lesions, 58
Renal function, in HIV patient, 20
Respiratory complaints of HIV-infected persons, 95, 106
Respiratory isolation with AFB isolation, comparison, 76

INDEX

Retrovir, 196–197. *See also* Zidovudine
Rifabutin, 26–27, 35, 190
   for MAC, 67
Rifadin, 190–191
Rifampin, 190–191
Rimactane, 190–191
Risk assessment, for HIV, 5–6. *See also* Testing for HIV infection
   benefits of learning HIV status, 6
   questions for, 6
Ritalin and Ritalin-SR, 180–181
2a-Roferon A, 161–162

Safer sex practices for HIV patient, 16
Sandostatin, 184
School for HIV-infected child, normal, 123
Seizures, of HIV-infected persons, 94, 103
Selenium deficiencies, 138
Septra, for *Pneumocystis carinii*, 24, 193–194
Serology, for diagnosis of *Coccidiomycosis*, 48–49
Serum cryptococcal antigen, 51
Sexually transmitted diseases, effectiveness of methods to prevent, 109–111
Shigella, drugs for, 189
Silvadene, 191–192
Silver sulfadiazine, 91, 191–192
   topical, 59
Sporanox, 177
Staphylococcus, drugs for, 191
Stavudine, 39–40, 192
   discussion, 39–40
   dosages, 40
   indications, 39
   monitoring, 40
   toxicity and side effects, 40
Steatosis, 35
Streptococcus, drugs for, 191
Streptomycin, 192–193
Sulfadiazine, 193
Supplementation
   anabolic agents, 139–140
   antioxidants, 138–139
   appetite stimulants, 139
   augmentation, 137–140
   nutritional, 137–140
   minerals, 138
   vitamins, 138
Symptomatic children, and frequency of follow-up, 125
Syphilis, 82–85
   diagnosis, 83
   presentation, 83
   treatment, 84–85

Testing considerations for HIV infection in children, 120–121
Testing for HIV infection
   posttest counseling, 8–9
   pretest counseling, 6–7
   prevention, 9–10
   risk assessment, 5–6
   tests, 8
Tetracyclnes, 37
Thrombocytopenia, 85–86
   diagnosis, 86
   presentation, 85–86
   treatment, 86
Thrombocytopenia purpura (ITP), in HIV patient, 20
TMP/SMX desensitization
   patient instructions for, 211
   for Pneumocystis carinii, 80
   protocol, 209
   as treatment for *Isospora belli*, 53
Toxoplasmosis, drugs for, 188
   with pyrimethamine, 193
Toxoplasmosis gondii, 28, 87–89
   diagnosis, 88
   presentation, 87
   treatment, 88–89
Toxoplasmosis encephalitis, medications for, 27–28
Training centers, AIDs, 217
Transmission of AIDs, prevention, 11
Trimethoprim/sulfamethoxazole (TMP/SMX), 193–194
   for *Pneumocystis carinii*, 24
Trimetrexate glucuronate, 194–195

Vaccines, for HIV-infected individuals, 159
Vaccines, viral, 197–200. *See also* Immunization
   influenza vaccine, 197–199
   pneumococcus vaccine, polyvalent, 199–200

INDEX

Varicella zoster, 90–92
  diagnosis, 91
  drugs for, 160
  immune globulin for HIV patient, 16
  presentation, 90
  treatment, 91–92
Velban, 195–196
Velsor, 195–196
Vesicular eruptions, 58
Videx, 36–38, 168–169. *See also* Didanosine
Vinblastine, intralesional, 195–196
Visceral protein or specific nutrient status of HIV-infected individual, 136
Vitamins, as nutritional supplementation, 138
VZV. *See* Varicella zoster

Wasting, patterns of, 134
Weight loss
  nutritional issues, 142
  patterns of, 134
  women and, 134
Wellcovorin, 174
Western blot test, 8
White people, number of AIDs cases among, 2
Women, HIV-infected
  cervical dysplasia and neoplasia, 111–112
  contraception techniques, 108
  gynecological concerns, 107–108
  gynecological infections, 108–111
  menstrual disorders, 111
  number of AIDs cases associated with, 1–2
  pregnancy in, 112–116
  recommendations, 107
  seropositive, screening of infants born to, 121–122
  and wasting, 134

Zalcitabine, 38–39, 114, 196
  discussions of indications, 38
  dosage, 39
  indications, 38
  monitoring, 39
  toxicity and side effects, 39
ZDV, see Zidovudine
Zerit, 39–40, 192. *See also* Stavudine
Zidovudine (ZDV), 21, 27, 34–36, 43, 196–197
  discussion, 34
  dosage, 34, 129
  for HIV-infected children, 120
  indications, 34, 129
  post-exposure, in health care workers, 153–155
  for pregnant woman, 114
  toxicity and side effects, 34–36, 129
Zinc deficiencies, 138
Zithromax, 165
Zovirax, 160, 161

COMMONLY USED MEDICATIONS FOR HIV/AIDS

Prophylaxis Against Opportunistic Infections:
- PCP (< 200 CD4 cells): TMP/SMX DS 1 tab QD or 3 times weekly **OR** dapsone 100 mg QD **OR** inhaled pentamidine 300 mg Q month (via Respirgard II nebulizer) **OR** 60 mg Q 2 weeks (via Fisoneb nebulizer, after loading dose)
- MAC (< 50 CD4 cells): Rifabutin 300 mg QD
- Toxoplasmosis (< 200 CD4 cells and toxoplasma serology positive): TMP/SMX DS QDor 3 times weekly **OR** dapsone 100 mg QD plus pyrimethamine 50 mg/week with folinic acid 25 mg/week

Antiretroviral Agents:
- Zidovudine: 200 mg TID (600 mg/day)
- Didanosine: > 60 kg—200 mg BID; < 60 kg—125 mg BID (each dose must include 2 chewable tablets; administer didanosine with or without zidovudine)
- Zalcitabine: 0.750 mg TID (with or without zidovudine)
- Stavudine: > 60 kg—40 mg BID; < 60 kg—30 mg BID

Candidiasis:
- Oral candida: Clotrimazole troches 10 mg dissolved orally 5 times daily **OR** nystatin 100,000 swish and swallow QID **OR** ketoconazole 200–400 mg 3 times weekly **OR** fluconazole 100 mg 3 times weekly
- Esophageal candida: Fluconazole 100–200 mg QD **OR** ketoconozole 200 mg BID for 4–21 days

Cryptococcus:
- Acute treatment: Amphotericin 0.5–1.0 mg/kg daily IV for 2–3 weeks, then fluconazole 400 mg QD for total of 8–12 weeks **OR** fluconazole 400–800 mg QD for 8–12 weeks
- Maintenance suppressive therapy: Fluconazole 200 mg QD for life

Cryptosporidium: Paromomycin 500–750 mg QID for 15–30 days, then 500 mg BID or antidiarrheal medications (see Diarrhea, below)

Cytomegalovirus: Gancyclovir (DHPG) 5 mg/kg BID IV induction for 1–21 days followed with 6 mg/kg IV QD 5 times weekly **OR** foscarnet 60 mg/kg Q 8 hours IV induction for 14–21 days followed with 90–120 mg/kg IV QD

Diarrhea: Loperamide 4 mg to start then 2 mg Q 6 hours or after each BM **OR** diaphenoxylate-atropine 2.5–5.0 mg TID **OR** tincture of opium 0.3–1.0 cc QID and PRN (max 6 cc/day)

Herpes Simplex:
- Acute treatment: Acyclovir 200 mg 5 times daily for 10–14 days
- Suppressive treatment: Acyclovir 200 mg TID or 400 mg BID
- Acyclovir-resistant herpes: Foscarnet

Herpes Zoster: Acyclovir 800 mg 5 times daily plus topical silver sulfadiazine for skin lesions. May require IV acyclovir

Mycobacterium avium Complex (MAC):
- Initial treatment: Clarithromycin 500 mg BID and clofazamine 100–200 mg QD with or without ethambutol 15–25 mg/kg/day. (Some experts recommend 3 drug therapy routinely.)
- If patient is acutely ill add amikacin 7.5 mg/kg/day IV or IM for 1–2 months
- If patient is intolerant or unresponsive to initial treatment, consider adding rifampin 300 mg/day or ciprofloxacin 750 mg BID

Mycobacterium tuberculosis:
- Positive PPD; history of positive PPD; anergy (in high risk patients): INH 300 mg QD with pyridoxine 50 mg QD for 12 months or more
- Active MTB: INH 300 mg QD plus rifampin 600 mg QD plus pyrazinamide 15–30 mg/kg QD plus either ethambutol 15–25 mg/kg QD or streptomycin 20 mg/kg QD. May discontinue ethambutol or streptomycin if indicated once sensitivities are available. Pyrazinamide may be discontinued after 2 months. Continue treatment for 9–12 months (or 6 months beyond culture conversion)
- **Directly observed therapy is recommended**

Peripheral Neuropathy: Amitriptyline 25–75 mg QD **OR** phenytoin 100 mg TID **OR** carbamazepine 100–300 mg BID **OR** capsaicin 0.075% cream QID topically

Pneumocystis Pneumonia: TMP/SMX 15 mg TMP/kg daily divided QID PO or IV **OR** pentamidine 4 mg/kg QD IV **OR** dapsone 100 mg QD (check G6PD level) plus TMP 15–20 mg/kg daily divided QID **OR** clindamycin 450 mg QID plus primaquine 30 mg QD **OR** atovaquone 750 mg PO TID with meals **OR** trimetrexate. Continue treatment for 21 days. Use adjunctive steroids $pO_2 < 70$ or Aa gradient > 35

Seborrheic Dermatitis: Hydrocortisone 2.5% cream (may add ketoconazole 2% cream BID)

Syphilis (> 1 year duration or neurosyphilis): Aqueous PCN G 2–4 MU Q 4 hours for 10 days **OR** procaine PCN G 2.4 MU IM QD plus probenecid 500 mg QID for 10 days. Consider PCN desensitization or ceftriaxone 1–2 g QD for 14 days in PCN-allergic patients

Toxoplasmosis*:
- Acute treatment: Sulfadiazine 75 mg/kg loading dose followed by 100 mg/kg/day (4–8 g divided BID–QID) plus pyrimethamine 100 mg QD for 2 days (loading dose) then 50–100 mg QD plus folinic acid 10–20 mg QD for at least 6–9 weeks
- Maintenance suppressive therapy: Sulfadiazine 2–4 g QD 3 times weekly plus pyrimethamine 50 mg QD 3 times weekly plus folinic acid. If patient is allergic to sulfa, substitute clindamycin 450 mg QID

* Sulfadiazine will prevent PCP in these patients. If sulfadiazine not available, call CDC (404) 488-4928

Weight Loss/Wasting: Dronabinol 25–10 mg BID **OR** megestrol 80–200 mg QID tablets or 800 mg/day suspension

---

From: Carmichael, Carmichael, & Fischl. *HIV/AIDS Primary Care Handbook*. Norwalk, CT: Appleton & Lange, © 1995.